HEART ATTACK DEMYSTIFIED

Heart Attack Myths Busted
Step-by-Step Guide to
Heart Attack Prevention and Care

Everyday Health Guide – Book 3

Dr. K. V. Sahasranam

Copyright

Copyright © 2024 by Sahasranam Kalpathy All rights reserved. No part of this book may be produced or stored in a retrieval system or transmitted in any form by any means, electronic, photocopying, recording, or otherwise, without express written permission of the author.

Disclaimer

The information in this book is intended for educational purposes only and is not a substitute for professional medical advice, diagnosis, or treatment. While every effort has been made to ensure accuracy, medical knowledge on heart attack continues to evolve, and readers should consult a healthcare provider for personalized advice when needed.

The patient scenarios included are fictional and meant for illustrative purposes. Some of these scenarios are from the author's own experience. But the names have been changed for preserving anonymity. Any treatments or lifestyle changes discussed should only be considered with professional medical guidance. The author and publishers are not liable for any loss or damage resulting from the use of this information.

*I dedicate this book
to my revered teachers of Medicine,
whose guidance instilled in me
the Art and Science of healing
and the wisdom to know when to intervene
and when to refrain.
My deepest gratitude and respects
are extended to each one of them.*

ॐ सर्वे भवन्तु सुखिन: सर्वे सन्तु निरामया: ।
सर्वे भद्राणि पश्यन्तु मा कश्चिद्दु:खभाग्भवेत् ।

**Om Sarve Bhavantu Sukhinah, Sarve Santu Niraamayaah |
Sarve Bhadraanni Pashyantu, Maa Kashcid-Duhkha-Bhaag-Bhavet |**

*Om, May All be Happy, May All be Free from Illness.
May All See what is Auspicious, May no one Suffer.*

A Humble Request to the Reader

Thank you for buying and reading this book. May I request your indulgence for one more favor.

I hope you enjoyed reading this book and derived benefit from the various topics discussed.

After reading the book, kindly give your sincere and valuable Review of this book in the Amazon site.

Your rating and candid review will be a great inspiration and encouragement to me.

Please check out my other books given at the end of this book.

Check out my Website at **kvsauthor.com**

You can contact me at my email address **kvsauthor@gmail.com**

TABLE OF CONTENTS

A Humble Request to the Reader 4
TABLE OF CONTENTS 5
Here's a Free Gift For You 11
About the Author 12
Author's Note 13
MORE BOOKS BY THE AUTHOR 14
Chapter 1: INTRODUCTION 15
Chapter 2: THE HISTORY OF HEART ATTACK 23
   Early References and Ancient Observations 23
   Rise of Electrocardiography (ECG) 26
   Coronary Angiography and Coronary Artery Revascularization 28
   Coronary Angioplasty and Modern Interventions 32
Chapter 3 HEART AND THE CIRCULATORY SYSTEM 33
   Structure and Function of the Circulatory System 33
   Pulmonary and Systemic Circulations 38
   The Coronary Arteries 38
Chapter 4 UNDERSTANDING CORONARY ARTERY DISEASE 42
   Role of Arteries in Heart Health 43
   Silent Coronary Artery Disease 45
   Sudden Cardiac Arrest Risk 46
   Coronary Artery Disease 46

Chapter 5 EPIDEMIOLOGY 52
   Prevalence and Incidence 52
   Global Burden 53
   Public Health Impact Of Heart Attack 59
   Why Heart Attacks Are More Common Today 60
      Changes in Diet 61
      Lifestyle Changes 62
Chapter 6 ANGINA PECTORIS 65
   What is Angina? 66
   Stable Angina 67
   Unstable Angina 69
   Symptoms of Angina 72
   Factors That Worsen Angina 75
   Management of Angina Pectoris 76
   Preventive Measures 78
Chapter 7 HEART ATTACK (MYOCARDIAL INFARCTION) 81
   What is a Heart Attack? 82
   Signs and Symptoms of a Heart Attack 85
Chapter 8 CAUSES OF HEART ATTACK 91
   How Blockages Form 92
   Coronary Artery Spasm 95
   Genetic (Inherited) Factors 97
Chapter 9 RISK FACTORS FOR HEART ATTACK 103
   Modifiable Risk Factors 105
   Non-Modifiable Risk Factors 115

Chapter 10 PATHOPHYSIOLOGY OF HEART ATTACK ... 118
   The Atherosclerotic Plaque ... 120
   Stable vs. Unstable Plaques ... 121
   Inflammation and Clot Formation ... 123
   Silent Heart Attack ... 126
Chapter 11 SYMPTOMS OF HEART ATTACK ... 129
   Common Symptoms ... 130
   Uncommon (Atypical) Symptoms ... 132
   Gender Difference in Symptoms ... 135
Chapter 12 DIAGNOSIS AND INVESTIGATIONS ... 139
   Tests Used in Diagnosis ... 140
   Imaging Tests ... 143
Chapter 13 PREHOSPITAL CARE OF HEART ATTACK ... 150
   Immediate Care ... 151
   Importance of Emergency Services ... 155
Chapter 14 EMERGENCY MANAGEMENT IN THE HOSPITAL ... 161
   Treatment in the Emergency Room ... 162
   Emergency Medications ... 166
   The Golden Hour ... 168
Chapter 15 FURTHER MANAGEMENT IN HOSPITAL ... 171
   Monitoring in the Intensive Care Unit ... 172
   Potential complications ... 174
   Medications to Prevent Future Heart Attacks ... 175
   Further Hospital Management ... 178
   Preparing the Patient for Discharge ... 181

Follow-Up Care 183
Chapter 16   COMPLICATIONS OF HEART ATTACK 186
   Acute Pulmonary Edema 187
   Chronic Heart Failure 191
   Mechanical Complications 193
   Ventricular Aneurysm 195
   Arrhythmias 197
   Cardiac Arrest 201
   Cardiogenic Shock 203
   Blood Clots 205
   Ischemic Cardiomyopathy (ICM) 210
   Pericardial Effusion 210
   Management of Complications 211
Chapter 17   CONVALESCENCE AFTER HEART ATTACK 216
   The Recovery Process 217
   Post-discharge care 218
   Changes in Lifestyle 223
   Emotional Recovery 228
Chapter 18   CARDIAC REHABILITATION 231
   What is Cardiac Rehabilitation? 232
   Key components of Cardiac Rehabilitation 233
   Psychological Support and Group Therapy 238
   Post-Heart Attack Medications 242
   Follow-Up 246
   Common Tests After a Heart Attack 247

Chapter 19 LIFESTYLE CHANGES AFTER HEART ATTACK 251
   A Heart-Healthy Diet 252
   Regular Exercise And Physical Activity 255
   Quitting Smoking 258
   Reducing Alcohol Intake 261
   Managing Stress 262
Chapter 20 PREVENTION HEART ATTACK 266
   Daily Habits That Lower Your Risk 267
   High Blood Pressure (Hypertension) 270
   High Blood Cholesterol 271
   Smoking and Alcohol Consumption 272
   Diabetes 272
   Obesity 273
   Other Chronic Conditions 274
   Public Health Campaigns & Prevention 275
Chapter 21 MISCELLANEOUS TOPICS 279
   Heart Attack and Pregnancy 280
   High Altitude Travel After a Heart Attack 285
   Air Travel After a Heart Attack 287
   Heart Attack After Non-Cardiac Surgery 289
Chapter 22 SUPPORT GROUPS AND RESOURCES 295
   Where to Find Support After a Heart Attack 296
   Governmental Resources 302
   Non-Governmental Resources 306

Chapter 23 THE FUTURE OF HEART ATTACK TREATMENT 312

   Biological Therapies... 313

   Gene Therapy and Its Potential 315

   New Drugs to Prevent Heart Damage and Recovery. 316

   Latest Advances in Prevention and Management 317

Chapter 24 CARDIAC ARREST AND CARDIOPULMONARY RESUSCITATION.. 320

   Cardiac Arrest 321

   Cardiopulmonary Resuscitation 322

   Step-by-Step CPR Guide 324

   Automated External Defibrillator 326

   Post-CPR Care.. 327

   Defibrillation 328

   YouTube Links for CPR 329

Resources & References... 332

   ACKNOWLEDGEMENT 341

Here's a Free Gift For You
Claim your **FREE** gift today!

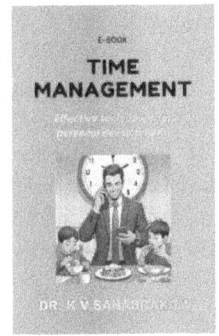

Unlock the secrets to mastering your time with *"Time Management - Mastering the Clock"*.

Learn how to spot and avoid common 'Time Wasters' that sneak into your day, so you can stay focused on what truly matters.

Don't miss this opportunity to take control of your schedule and start achieving your goals more efficiently!

Get your FREE eBook now. VISIT THE SITE Below

https://sahasranam.ck.page/68c54bb5e5

Or SCAN The QR Code given below

About the Author

Dr. K. V. Sahasranam MD, DM, FACC, FCSI, is a distinguished Cardiologist and former Professor of Cardiology at Calicut Medical College, India. With over 45 years of medical practice, he has retired and now resides in the USA. His deep passion lies in educating students and residents, reflected in his book, "**Understanding the Electrocardiogram**," designed for medical students and physicians, which thoroughly explores the ECG and simplifies its interpretation. Additionally, Dr. Sahasranam offers a comprehensive *3-module course on ECG* through the **Udemy.com** platform.

Writing under the pen name *'Sahasranam Kalpathy,'* he has authored 12 more books, spanning both fiction and nonfiction. His works include a series on *'Problems of the Elderly'* (2 books), *'Understanding Hinduism'* (3 books), *'Skillsets for Success'* (2 books), three captivating Fiction novels and two books of Short stories for children.

His first book in the *'Everyday Health Guide'* series' is titled "***Diabetes Demystified***". The second book in the series is "***High Blood Pressure Demystified***". This is the third book in the series.

Visit his WEBSITE at: **kvsauthor.com**

Or SCAN the QR code below

Author's Note

Having written two books in the *"Everyday Health Guide"* series, I felt it was important to bring attention to the serious condition of heart attacks. My first two books, *"Diabetes Demystified"* and *"High Blood Pressure Demystified"*, offered comprehensive discussions on those conditions in considerable detail.

Encouraged by the feedback from colleagues and readers, I decided to write a third book on Heart Attacks, as this issue has become a growing threat in today's world. In the past, I have heard my father often say that heart attacks were primarily a disease of the elderly and the affluent, with younger generations and those from lower socioeconomic backgrounds rarely affected. Unfortunately, this is no longer the case. Over the course of my long career, first in a medical college and later in a multispecialty corporate hospital, I witnessed heart attacks affecting people from all walks of life, including younger individuals.

One of the most distressing cases involved a 19-year-old medical student who died of a heart attack while studying for exams in his college hostel. He was rushed to the emergency room, where it was discovered that he had suffered a massive heart attack. This happened before coronary angiography and angioplasty were widely available.

As society evolves, modernization has brought with it numerous challenges. One of the most significant consequences is the rise of "Lifestyle Diseases," with heart attacks leading the charge. It is with this in mind that I found it necessary to discuss the various aspects of this formidable condition in a way that is easily understandable for readers.

With these few words I present this book to you.

Dr. K. V. Sahasranam MD, DM (Cardiology) FACC.

MORE BOOKS BY THE AUTHOR

NON-FICTION

How to Face the Challenges while Growing Old — Problems of Elderly Book 1

Old Age Health Challenges and Solutions — Problems of Elderly Book 2

Understanding the Electrocardiogram — Medical Book on ECG

Demystifying Hinduism — Understanding Hinduism Book 1

The Avadhoota – Whispers of Wisdom — Understanding Hinduism Book 2

Daily Musings — Understanding Hinduism Book 3

How to Master Essential Life Skills - Skill sets for Success Book 1

How to Achieve Professional Excellence - Skill sets for Success Book 2

FICTION

Tell Me a Story, Grandpa - Short Stories for Children Book 1

Grandpa, Tell me More Stories — Short Stories for Children-2

In Search of a Bridegroom — An Autobiographical Fiction

The Truth Lies Out There - A Family Drama of Suspense

Code Black - A Hospital based Thriller

Diabetes Demystified - Everyday Health Guide Book 1

High Blood Pressure Demystified — Everyday Health Guide Book 2

Chapter 1: INTRODUCTION

A heart attack, also known as *"Myocardial Infarction"* (**MI**), is a serious medical emergency that occurs when the blood flow to a part of the heart is blocked. This blockage prevents oxygen and nutrients from reaching the heart muscle, causing damage to the affected part. In simple terms, the heart is a pump that continuously needs oxygen-rich blood to keep working, just like any other muscle in our body. When this supply is interrupted, even for a few minutes, the heart muscle begins to suffer and can eventually die if the flow is not restored quickly.

Understanding what a heart attack is and how it happens is crucial. Many people may not fully comprehend the dangers of this condition or how easily it can occur. It is not just something that happens suddenly without warning. The buildup of fatty deposits (*plaque*) in the arteries over time restricts blood flow and sets the stage for a heart attack. This process is called *"Atherosclerosis"* (hardening and narrowing of the arteries), and it develops over years due to factors such as poor diet, lack of exercise, smoking, and stress – to name a few. Knowing this can help people take steps to prevent it from happening.

Heart attacks are one of the leading causes of death worldwide. However, they are preventable in many cases, and understanding the risks and symptoms can make a significant difference in reducing the chances of experiencing one. That is why learning about heart attacks, their symptoms, causes, and prevention is incredibly important for everyone, regardless of age or health status.

Some Important Technical Terms

Before proceeding further, let us briefly get acquainted with some terms used in this book which are derived from medical terminology.

__Metabolism refers to the physical and chemical reactions in the body that change food into energy and those that use energy__. They are the sum total of all chemical changes that take place in a cell or an organism. These changes generate energy and produce many other chemical substances that the cells and organisms need to grow, reproduce, and stay healthy. Metabolism also helps get rid of toxic substances from the body by destroying them mainly in the liver.

__Homeostasis refers to any automatic process that a living being uses to keep its body steady on the inside while continuing to adjust to conditions outside of the body, or in its environment__. The body makes these changes constantly to work and survive. A state of balance among all the body systems is needed for the body to survive and function correctly. *__Homeostasis is the ability to maintain a relatively stable internal state that persists despite changes in the world outside.__* For example, whether the surrounding temperature rises or falls, the human body remarkably maintains its internal temperature at a steady 37 degrees Celsius (98.6 degrees Fahrenheit). Similarly, the pH of blood is tightly regulated within the range of 7.35 to 7.45, ensuring the stability necessary for vital biochemical processes to occur seamlessly.

Mortality means the rate of death, or the number of deaths occurring in a specific population over a given period of time. It refers to how many people die from a particular disease or condition. In other words, it means the death rate, or the number of deaths in a certain group of people in a certain period of time. Mortality may be reported for people who have a certain disease, live in one area of the country, or who are of a certain gender, age, or ethnic group. Doctors and researchers might discuss the *"mortality rate"* of a disease, meaning how likely someone is to die from that disease.

Morbidity refers to a disease or medical condition that causes illness or injury but does not result in death. It can also refer to the negative effects of a medical treatment or surgery. The physical and psychological impact of a chronic condition, such as decreased quality of life or chronic symptoms is also called *morbidity* due to that condition. It is the amount of disease within a population. *Medical problems caused by a treatment is also referred to as morbidity.*

Prognosis in medical terms means a doctor's prediction about how a disease is likely to develop and what the chances of recovery are for a patient, essentially it is a "forecast" of what to expect with an illness. It is the likely outcome or course of a disease, the chance of recovery or recurrence. A prognosis is based on the doctor's knowledge of the disease and the patient's individual situation, but it need not always be completely accurate. When giving a prognosis, a doctor will consider things like the severity of the disease, the patient's age and overall health, and the available treatment options. Hence, it indicates the likely outcome or course of the disease - the chance of recovery or recurrence or death.

Body Mass Index (BMI) is a measure of body fat based on the height and weight of a person. It is applicable for adults.

BMI is calculated by dividing the weight (in kilograms) by the square of the height (in meters). It can also be calculated by dividing the weight in pounds by the square of the height in inches multiplied by a conversion faction of 703.

$$\text{BMI} = \frac{\text{Weight (in Kg)}}{\text{Height (in meters)}^2}$$

$$\text{BMI} = \left[\frac{\text{Weight (in pounds)}}{\text{(Height (in inches)}^2}\right] \times 703$$

An easy rule of thumb to determine your ideal weight is as follows - subtract 100 from your height in centimeters. The result is your ideal weight in kilograms. For instance, if your height is 160 centimeters (5'4"), your ideal weight would be 160 minus 100, which equals 60 kilograms.

Inflammation is a normal part of the body's immune response to injury or infection. It is a process that involves the release of chemicals that trigger the body to fight off infection or heal damaged tissue. It is the body's immune system's response to an irritant, injury or infection. Inflammation can be caused by a number of factors, including trauma, invasion by bacteria or viruses, noxious compounds, toxic chemicals, foreign bodies like a thorn and environmental agents.

Symptoms of inflammation include pain, redness, heat, swelling, and loss of function. While inflammation can be a normal and healthy part of the body's response to injury, it can also harm health if it occurs in healthy tissues or goes on for too long.

What Is The Purpose Of This Book?

This book is written with one simple goal in mind: to make the complex world of heart attacks easy to understand for everyone. Medical terminology and explanations can often be overwhelming for people without a background in healthcare. However, understanding your own health is the first step towards taking control of it.

The purpose of this book is to break down the critical aspects of heart attacks, from what causes them to how they can be prevented and managed. By simplifying medical concepts, this book aims to empower readers to make informed decisions about their health. Whether you, or a loved one has had a heart attack, or you are simply looking to prevent one, this book will provide you with the knowledge and tools to understand the condition better.

Throughout this book, we will explore various topics related to heart attacks, including lifestyle changes, medications, and other treatments that can help manage or prevent heart disease. You will also find practical advice and tips to help you make healthier choices in your daily life, such as improving your diet, increasing physical activity, and reducing stress.

For those living with a heart attack, this book will offer guidance on recovery and long-term care, emphasizing the importance of following medical advice and making necessary lifestyle adjustments to reduce the risk of future heart problems. One whole chapter is dedicated to the prevention of heart attack.

One unique aspect which readers will note about this book is that certain important points about heart attacks will be repeated across different chapters. This repetition is *intentional*. It ensures that readers, even if they choose to read only certain sections, will still receive all the critical information needed for a complete understanding of heart attacks. Each chapter is designed to stand on its own, so readers can explore specific topics without having to follow the book in sequence. This format is meant to accommodate both casual readers and those seeking comprehensive knowledge.

The three chapters—*Convalescence After Heart Attack, Cardiac Rehabilitation*, and *Lifestyle After Heart Attack*—share common themes, such as exercise and diet. Readers may question the repetition, but each chapter offers subtle nuances and distinct information. Therefore, readers are kindly requested not to be concerned by the overlap in content.

To further aid in understanding, medical terms will be explained clearly within the text itself, often with definitions provided in parentheses. This approach ensures that even if unfamiliar terminology is used, it is immediately clarified, making the information more accessible. You won't need to flip to a glossary or feel confused by unfamiliar words.

Certain sentences, particularly definitions, are italicized and gently underlined with dotted lines to highlight key points and capture the reader's attention. This subtle emphasis helps important information to stand out, making it easier for readers to focus on the most critical details.

Each chapter will start with a brief introductory paragraph, giving a brief overview of the key points covered. This way, you can get a sense of what the chapter will focus on before diving into the details. At the end of each chapter, you will also find "*Key Takeaways,*" which summarize the most important facts and ideas discussed.

In addition to scientific discussions, the book will include patient stories that illustrate real-life experiences with heart attacks. These stories are based on the author's medical practice, though the names and details have been changed to protect privacy. By sharing these personal experiences, the book aims to provide practical insights into how heart attacks can affect individuals and families, and how people can manage the condition in their everyday lives.

Throughout this book, I have included many images to emphasize that a picture is worth a thousand words and to make reading more engaging. Most of these images were sourced from depositphotos.com, and I am deeply grateful to them for providing such excellent visuals. Some of the images were created using AI tools available through designer.microsoft.com. The ECGs featured in the book are from my personal collection, gathered over many years of medical practice.

Lastly, towards the end of the book, you will find chapters dedicated to resources, support groups, and helpful apps that can make managing heart disease easier. The penultimate chapter will explore the future of heart attack management, discussing potential advancements in treatments and emerging technologies that could shape the care of tomorrow.

The final chapter of the book on '*Cardiopulmonary Resuscitation*' (**CPR**) aims to acquaint the reader with the CPR technique and provide a concise overview of how it is performed. This knowledge can be vital in emergency situations, particularly when someone experiences a sudden cardiac arrest. If a trained individual is nearby, performing CPR could potentially save a life. *Readers are urged to learn this technique through reputable sources, and a few links demonstrating the procedure have been included for further guidance.*

In conclusion, this book is not only a guide for those who have experienced a heart attack but also for individuals who want to take proactive steps in preventing one. By empowering readers with knowledge, this book seeks to contribute to the fight against heart disease, helping to reduce the number of heart attacks and improving the quality of life for those affected by them.

Chapter 2: THE HISTORY OF HEART ATTACK

Heart attacks, a leading cause of death worldwide for over three decades, are not merely a modern affliction but have roots tracing back to ancient history. Over time, medical practitioners and researchers, from ancient Egyptian physicians to modern cardiologists, have contributed to understanding, diagnosing, and treating cardiovascular disease. This chapter explores the major milestones in the history of heart attacks, uncovering both ancient insights and modern innovations.

Early References and Ancient Observations
The Egyptians and Early Medical Records

The ancient Egyptians, as early as 3000 BC, were advanced in medicine, often studying symptoms now recognized as related to heart disease. The *"Ebers Papyrus"*, an ancient Egyptian medical text, contains descriptions that resemble angina pectoris, where pain radiates to the arms, chest, and sides, ominously warning that *"…….And if though examinst a man for illness in his cardia, suffering from pain in the arms, the breast, and in the side of his cardia………… it is death that threatens him."* Homer's *"Odyssey"* also references the Egyptians' medical prowess, noting that they were *"skilled in medicine more than any other art."*

In recent years, evidence of atherosclerosis—a condition that leads to heart attacks—was discovered in Egyptian mummies from 3000 years ago. In 2013, the Lancet published a study showing that CT scans of mummies revealed atherosclerotic plaques in about a third of the 137 specimens, suggesting that this disease was present even among ancient populations.

Early Greek Contributions

Greek physicians, too, were pioneers in medical observations. They conducted dissections, which likely provided early understandings of bodily organs and the circulatory system. By the 15th century, Leonardo da Vinci, the renowned Italian polymath, observed that with age, blood vessels thicken, limiting blood flow. He stated that *"vessels in the elderly restrict the transit of blood through thickening of the tunics."* This recognition of vascular change hinted at the process leading to heart disease and helped lay the groundwork for later anatomical studies.

Medical Advances in Europe and the Modern Understanding of Angina

In 1768, English physician William Heberden presented a landmark paper, *"Some Account of a Disorder of the Breast,"* before the Royal College of Physicians London in 1768, describing the condition now recognized as *Angina Pectoris*. Heberden noted that his patients experienced intense, crushing chest pain while walking, especially after meals, which would dissipate upon rest. He coined the term *"Angina Pectoris,"* with *"angina"* meaning 'strangling' in Greek and *"pectoris"* translating to 'chest' in Latin. His description given below remains one of the most vivid early accounts of this condition.

> *"Those who are afflicted with it are seized, while they are walking, and more particularly when they walk soon after eating, with a painful and most disagreeable sensation in the breast, which seems as if it would take their life away, if it were to increase or to continue: The moment they stand still, all this uneasiness vanishes."*

Giovanni Morgagni, an Italian anatomist, described atherosclerosis as *"hardening of the arteries"* in 1761. His observations were instrumental in understanding how arteries can become rigid due to plaque buildup, leading to restricted blood flow—a key factor in heart disease.

Rudolf Virchow, known as the 'father of Pathology,' studied the formation of blood clots, or thrombosis, within the arteries and veins, identifying factors that predispose blood vessels to such blockages. His work provided critical insights into the mechanisms of coronary thrombosis, a major cause of heart attacks.

Animal Experiments

By the late 19th century, experiments with dogs demonstrated that tying off the coronary arteries led to ventricular fibrillation—a condition in which the heart's ventricles "quiver" instead of beating effectively—resulting in the animal's death. These findings were a breakthrough in understanding how blocked coronary arteries could lead to fatal outcomes in humans.

Cardiac Catheterization

In the 19th century, Claude Bernard pioneered cardiac catheterization by introducing glass tubes into the blood vessels of horses to measure pressure in the heart chambers. Building on this, Werner Forssman in 1929 performed the first human cardiac catheterization on himself, paving the way for further studies. His work inspired André Frédéric Cournand and Dickinson Richards, who refined the procedure, leading to their joint Nobel Prize in 1956.

Rise of Electrocardiography (ECG)

The *Electrocardiogram* (**ECG**) revolutionized the diagnosis of heart diseases in the early twentieth century. It was Augustus Waller who in 1887 first recorded and demonstrated the ECG of the human heart. He was a British physiologist in London. But at that time, he did not recognize the importance of this discovery. Willem Einthoven, who was a witness to this demonstration by

Waller was inspired by this and took up the challenge to develop this further.

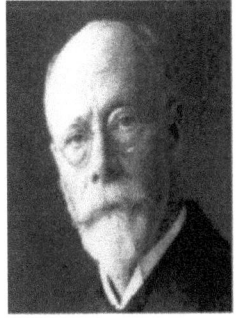

Thus, it was Willem Einthoven (1860-1927), a Dutch physiologist, who took this idea forward and recorded the ECG using a string galvanometer. It was he who named it the '*Electrocardiogram*'. He named the deflections "P-QRS-T-U" and published his findings in 1902. His ECG tracing was of fairly good

Willem Einthoven
(Courtesy: Hulton Archive/Getty Images)

quality. In 1905 he presented cases of atrial and ventricular hypertrophy, ventricular bigeminy, ventricular premature beats and identified the 'U' wave in the ECG. The same year, he transmitted the ECG via telephone and recorded it 1500 meters away. Einthoven's electrocardiograph which recorded the first ECG weighed 600 lbs.

In 1924, Einthoven was awarded the Nobel prize in Physiology and Medicine "*For the discovery of the mechanism of the electrocardiogram*". Initially, his recording had only three leads. Einthoven conceived the famous *Einthoven's Equilateral Triangle* with these three leads. which facilitates electrical axis calculation.

The invention of the ECG machine revolutionized the diagnosis of heart attacks and subsequently refinements in the ECG machine reduced its size and made bedside diagnosis of heart diseases easy.

Coronary Angiography and Coronary Artery Revascularization

In 1958, Dr. Mason Jones unintentionally performed the first coronary angiogram while doing cardiac catheterization, when a catheter entered a coronary artery by accident. Realizing the diagnostic potential, physicians like Dr. Judkins and Dr. Amplatz refined this technique, making coronary angiography a standard procedure for diagnosing coronary artery disease.

One of the significant developments facilitating coronary artery bypass surgery was the coronary arteriogram, a diagnostic imaging technique. This test provides a detailed image of the coronary arteries, allowing surgeons to pinpoint areas of blockage. The coronary arteriogram made it possible to map out treatment strategies and determine the necessity for surgical intervention in patients with CAD. It provided an essential foundation for planning revascularization procedures and significantly improved the diagnosis and management of coronary artery disease.

Coronary Artery Bypass Grafting (CABG)

One of the most effective treatments for severe CAD is coronary artery bypass grafting (**CABG**), a surgical technique developed over the course of the 20th century..

The roots of coronary artery revascularization trace back to the pioneering work of Alexis Carrel in 1910. Carrel, a French surgeon, developed and refined surgical techniques in animal models, specifically dogs, that closely resemble modern CABG. His experiments involved suturing and connecting blood vessels, an approach essential to modern revascularization procedures. Carrel's work earned him a Nobel Prize in 1912 and laid the groundwork for later surgical advancements in heart and vascular surgery.

In 1961, Dr. Robert Goetz performed what is widely considered the first coronary artery bypass procedure in a human. Though rudimentary by today's standards, Goetz's operation marked the beginning of bypass surgery as a viable option for treating blocked coronary arteries. This procedure connected a vessel from another part of the body to the coronary artery, enabling blood to bypass the blocked section and restore blood flow to the heart muscle.

The Heart-Lung Machine and Its Role in CABG

A key technological innovation enabling more complex cardiac surgeries was the development of the heart-lung machine by Dr. John Gibbon in 1954. Originally designed to repair congenital heart defects, this device temporarily took over the function of the heart and lungs during surgery, maintaining blood circulation and oxygenation in the body. By freeing surgeons from the immediate risk of heart stoppage, the heart-lung machine made it possible to operate on the heart with greater precision and duration. This technology quickly became a staple in coronary artery bypass grafting procedures, facilitating safe and effective revascularization surgery.

The Rise of Modern CABG

In 1967, Dr. René G. Favaloro performed what is considered the first modern coronary artery bypass graft surgery at the Cleveland Clinic. His approach involved using a section of the saphenous vein, taken from the patient's leg, to create a bypass around the blocked section of the coronary artery. Favaloro's technique offered a more reliable and durable solution for patients with multiple coronary obstructions. This method rapidly gained popularity and set the standard for future bypass surgeries.

By the 1960s, coronary artery bypass grafting had matured into a standardized surgical technique, becoming a routine procedure in treating severe coronary artery disease. The reliability of CABG as a treatment option allowed it to be performed widely in medical centers across the world. The procedure proved especially beneficial for individuals with multiple blocked arteries, as it could alleviate symptoms of angina, reduce the risk of heart attacks, and improve heart function. As the success rates and safety of the surgery increased, CABG became one of the mainstays in the treatment of CAD.

The introduction of CABG provided a lifesaving option for patients with advanced or complex forms of coronary artery disease that were not manageable through lifestyle changes or medication alone. CABG is particularly effective for patients with multi-vessel disease, where several arteries are obstructed, making the heart's oxygen supply insufficient to meet its demands. By bypassing these blockages, CABG helps restore adequate blood flow, improving the heart's efficiency and reducing symptoms like chest pain and fatigue.

CABG has been shown to improve the quality of life and prognosis for heart patients, effectively reducing symptoms like chest pain and shortness of breath. In patients with severe CAD, it can prevent further heart attacks, improve exercise tolerance, and even extend life expectancy. CABG is now performed in hundreds of thousands of patients annually, proving its importance and effectiveness as a treatment for CAD. Advances in surgical techniques and post-operative care have also contributed to improved survival rates and outcomes for patients undergoing the procedure.

Since the inception of CABG, the field of cardiac surgery has seen continuous advancements, further refining the original technique. Innovations such as minimally invasive CABG, where smaller incisions are used, and off-pump CABG, where surgery is performed on a beating heart without the heart-lung machine, have been developed. These methods reduce recovery time and complications, offering additional options for suitable candidates and reflecting the ongoing evolution of coronary surgery.

The history of coronary artery bypass grafting is a testament to the power of medical innovation in improving patient care and outcomes.

The Concept of Coronary Care Units (CCUs)

In 1961, Dr. Desmond Julian introduced the concept of *Coronary Care Units* (**CCUs**) at the Royal Infirmary in Edinburgh. His approach emphasized continuous cardiac monitoring, closed chest massage, and emergency protocols to improve the survival rates of heart attack patients. This model transformed emergency cardiac care, enabling swift and effective responses during acute events. The CCUs have helped to bring down the mortality rates in heart attacks.

Coronary Angioplasty and Modern Interventions

In 1977, Andreas Gruentzig performed the first coronary angioplasty, a minimally invasive procedure using a balloon-tipped catheter to compress arterial plaque. This technique rapidly evolved, leading to stents and more sophisticated devices to keep arteries open, representing a monumental shift in the treatment of coronary artery disease.

The journey from early observations of heart pain in ancient Egypt to today's advanced diagnostic and surgical techniques tells a fascinating story of human ingenuity and medical progress. Each step—from Heberden's description of angina to Einthoven's ECG and Forssman's catheterization—has contributed to understanding and managing heart disease more effectively. Modern medicine, through innovations like CABG, coronary angiography, and angioplasty, has reshaped heart attack treatment, saving countless lives. The historical progression of these discoveries highlights our evolving battle with heart disease, underscoring the critical role of past breakthroughs in shaping today's healthcare.

Chapter 3 HEART AND THE CIRCULATORY SYSTEM

Before considering the specifics of coronary artery disease and heart attack, it is important to understand the heart and the circulatory system, as these are at the core of the body's blood circulation and blood pressure regulation.

Structure and Function of the Circulatory System

The circulatory system's primary role is to deliver blood to various parts of the body, ensuring the supply of oxygen and nutrients while removing waste products. The heart, a remarkable muscular organ, lies at the center of this system. Despite its small size—approximately that of a closed fist, weighing around 9-12 ounces (250-350 grams)—the heart pumps blood throughout the body, operating tirelessly throughout one's life.

The Chambers of the Heart

Located slightly to the left inside the chest cavity, the heart is shielded by the breastbone in front and spine behind. It contains four chambers - two upper chambers known as the *Atria* (singular: *Atrium*) and two lower chambers called the *Ventricles*. The atria receive blood from all parts of the body, while the ventricles pump it out.

Blood enters the right atrium (**RA**) from two large veins: the *Superior Vena Cava* (**SVC**), which collects blood from the upper body, and the Inferior Vena Cava (**IVC**), which collects blood from the lower body. On the left side, oxygenated blood from the lungs enters the *Left Atrium* (**LA**) via four *Pulmonary Veins* – two from each lung. From the LA blood enters the *Left Ventricle* (**LV**) which pumps this oxygen-rich blood into the *Aorta*, the body's largest artery. The aorta distributes the blood to the rest of the body through its various branches. Meanwhile, the *Right Ventricle* (**RV**) pumps *deoxygenated* (oxygen-poor) blood into the *Pulmonary Artery*, which carries it to the lungs for oxygenation. [**Fig 3. 1**]

Arteries, Veins, and Capillaries

Blood vessels play a vital role in the process of circulation. Arteries, such as the aorta, transport oxygen-rich blood from the heart to various parts of the body. The walls of the arteries contain smooth muscles that allow vessels to expand or widen (*dilate*) and contract or narrow (*constrict*) as blood flows through them. In contrast, veins return oxygen-poor, carbon dioxide-rich blood back to the heart. Once in the lungs, oxygen from the air we breathe in is absorbed into the blood, while carbon dioxide is expelled as we exhale.

The inner lining of the arteries and veins are composed of a sheet of cells called the *Endothelium*. The endothelium releases a protein called *Endothelin* which caused blood vessels to become narrow (*constrict*).

As arteries move away from the heart, they branch into increasingly smaller vessels, culminating in tiny *Capillaries*. These hair-thin vessels have walls so thin that oxygen and nutrients can pass into the surrounding tissues, while carbon dioxide and metabolic waste move from the tissues into the blood. The capillaries then converge into veins, which carry the waste-laden blood back to the heart. This circulation cycle ensures the continuous distribution and exchange of vital substances throughout the body.

Heart Valves: Ensuring One-Way Blood Flow

Within the heart, blood flows only in one direction, thanks to a system of valves that act like gates. Between the atria and ventricles are two main valves: the *Tricuspid Valve* (**TV**) on the right side, and the *Mitral Valve* (**MV**) on the left side. These prevent backflow of blood into the atria. Similarly, the *Aortic Valve* (**AV**) and *Pulmonary Valve* (**PV**) prevent blood from flowing back into the ventricles after being pumped out to the body or lungs through the aorta and the pulmonary artery respectively. This system ensures a smooth, forward flow of blood through the heart and circulatory system. **[Fig 3. 1]**

The Heartbeat: The Body's Electrical System

The heart beats around 70 times per minute in a healthy adult, thanks to a small but vital structure called the *Sinus Node* (**SA**). This node is located in the upper right chamber of the heart (*right atrium*) and acts like a natural pacemaker or generator, sending out regular electrical signals (*impulse*) that tell the heart when to beat. These signals travel through special pathways in the heart, like the wiring in the walls of a building, making the heart muscles contract together in rhythm.

After starting in the Sinus Node, the *impulse* moves down to another group of cells called the *Atrio-Ventricular* (**AV**) *Node*, which is found between the upper and lower chambers of the heart. The AV Node works like a control switch, briefly delaying the signal so the upper chambers have time to pump all the blood into the lower chambers. Once the signal passes through the AV node, it makes the lower chambers contract, sending blood to the lungs and the rest of the body.

From the AV Node, the signal travels along two main paths, called the Right and Left Bundle branches, which go to the lower chambers of the heart. The left branch splits into smaller branches that reach deep into the left lower chamber (*left ventricle*). These spread out like the branches of a tree and end in tiny fibers called *Purkinje fibers*. These fibers carry the electrical impulse to the heart muscle, making it contract and keep the heart beating.

The heart works continuously throughout life, with only brief milliseconds of rest between beats. Remarkably, it beats about 100,000 times each day—an incredible testament to its endurance.

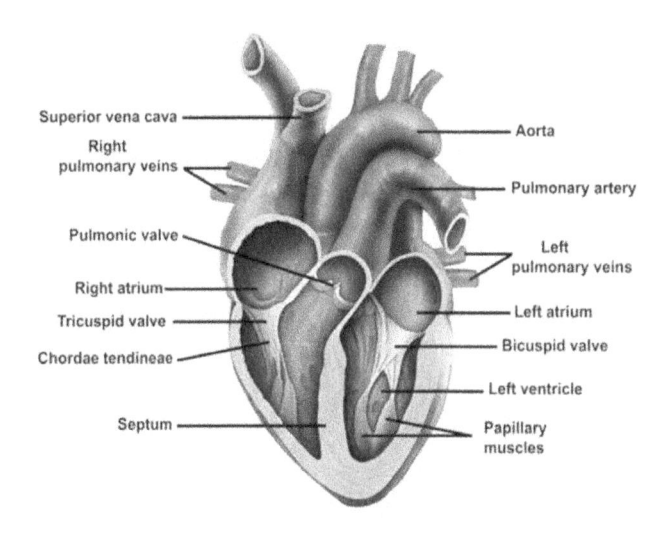

Fig 3. 1. Structure of the Heart

The figure showing the internal structure of the heart with the cardiac chambers, great vessels, veins and valves.

(Courtesy: Vishmaya88 / Depositphotos.com)

The Heart's Vital Role

The heart's primary function is to pump oxygen-rich blood to every part of the body, while also collecting carbon dioxide and waste products. The carbon dioxide is expelled through the lungs during exhalation, and the waste products are filtered out by the kidneys and excreted as urine or processed by the liver and eliminated from the body. The heart also plays a critical role in maintaining the body's blood pressure, pumping approximately 5.5 liters (1.5 gallons) of blood every minute in an adult.

Despite its relentless work, the heart requires its own supply of oxygen and nutrients. This is delivered via three small arteries, called the *Coronary Arteries*, which arise from the aorta and encircle the heart. A blockage in these arteries can lead to a heart attack, one of the most serious cardiovascular events.

Pulmonary and Systemic Circulations

The circulatory system is divided into two circuits: *Pulmonary Circulation* and *Systemic Circulation*. **[Fig 3. 2]**

Pulmonary Circulation: Blood enters the right ventricle from the superior and inferior vena cava, and is pumped into the pulmonary artery, which transports it to the lungs. There, the blood is oxygenated before returning to the left atrium via the pulmonary veins. This short loop of circulation, responsible for oxygenating blood, is referred to as the '*Lesser circulation.*'

Systemic Circulation: Oxygenated blood from the left ventricle enters the aorta and is carried throughout the body via its numerous branches. As blood flows through organs and tissues, it delivers oxygen and nutrients, collecting carbon dioxide and waste products in return. This deoxygenated blood is then brought back to the right atrium by the superior and inferior vena cava. This much longer route is known as the '*Greater circulation.*'

The Coronary Arteries

The heart itself needs blood to stay healthy and do its job supplying it with oxygen and nutrients. Two main arteries supply blood to the heart: the *Left Main*

Coronary Artery (**LMCA**) and the *Right Coronary Artery* (**RCA**). These arise from the aorta near its origin from the left ventricle.

The *Left Main Coronary Artery* (**LMCA**) splits further into two branches:

- The *Left Anterior Descending* (**LAD**) Artery which supplies blood to the front of the heart.

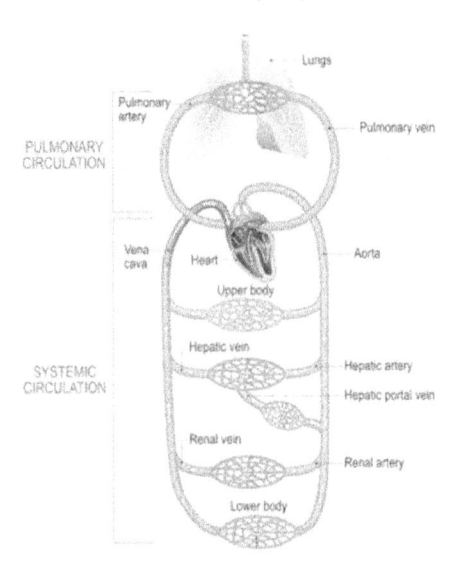

Fig 3. 2. Pulmonary & Systemic Circulation

The figure showing the Pulmonary and Systemic Circulations.

(Courtesy: Edesignua /Depositphotos.com)

- The *Left Circumflex Artery* (**LCX**) which supplies blood to the sides and back of the heart.

The *Right Coronary Artery* (**RCA**) supplies blood to the right side of the heart and the under surface of the left side.

Veins on the surface of the heart collect the used blood and return it to the right atrium through a large vein called the *Coronary Sinus*. Some smaller veins, called *Thebesian Veins*, also help drain blood from the heart.

Without proper blood flow through these arteries, the heart muscle cannot function effectively, potentially leading to heart disease.

Some Fascinating Facts about the heart

- *The human heart is about the size of the individual's closed fist.*
- *It beats around 100,000 times per day.*
- *The average adult heart beats 60-100 times per minute, while a newborn's heart beats much faster at 100-160 beats per minute.*
- *The heart has its own electrical conduction system that coordinates the contractions of the different chambers. This system includes the sinoatrial (SA) node, which acts as the heart's natural pacemaker.*
- *The heart pumps about 1.5 gallons (5.5 liters)of blood per minute, amounting to over 2,000 gallons per day. Over an average lifetime, the heart will pump around 1 million barrels of blood.*

- *During strenuous exercise, the heart can pump up to 5-7 times more blood than when the body is at rest.*
- *Blood travels about 12,000 miles throughout the body daily—roughly four times the distance across the United States.*
- *The body contains approximately 60,000 miles (96,560 km) of blood vessels, enough to circle the Earth twice.*
- *The heart creates enough pressure to squirt blood 30 feet (9 meters).*

By understanding the heart and circulatory system, we gain insight into how blood pressure is regulated and how it affects the health of these vital structures.

Chapter 4 UNDERSTANDING CORONARY ARTERY DISEASE

Coronary Artery Disease (CAD) is one of the most common and dangerous heart conditions, affecting millions of people worldwide. It occurs when the arteries that supply blood to the heart become narrowed or blocked due to plaque buildup, restricting blood flow and putting individuals at risk for heart attacks. Often developing silently over years, CAD can go unnoticed until serious complications arise. Understanding the causes and symptoms of CAD is vital for early detection and prevention. This chapter is designed to educate readers generally on how CAD develops, its risk factors, and how to recognize warning signs like chest pain or angina.

Coronary Artery Disease (**CAD**) is one of the most common heart conditions worldwide. CAD affects millions of people globally. It is one of the leading causes of heart attacks around the world. It is a condition where the arteries, which supply blood to the heart, become damaged or blocked. Understanding how this happens and what causes it is key to protecting your heart health and reducing the risk of serious complications like a heart attack. Understanding how this condition develops and why it can be so dangerous is crucial for preventing serious heart problems.

Hence, understanding the basics of CAD is the first step towards protecting your heart. *Cardiovascular Disease (**CVD**) is a broad term encompassing any disease affecting the heart or blood vessels, while Coronary Artery Disease (**CAD**) is a specific type of CVD that refers to the narrowing or blockage of the coronary arteries which supply blood to the heart muscle.* It is usually caused by plaque buildup within the artery wall. Essentially, CAD is a heart disease within the larger category of CVDs.

The word *'cardiac'* means *'relating to, or affected by, the heart'*. The root of the word is the Ancient Greek word *kardiá*, which means "heart".

Role of Arteries in Heart Health

To better understand CAD, it helps to first think of the arteries as the body's highways. Just as roads transport goods and supplies to different places, arteries transport essential oxygen and nutrients to the different parts of the body keeping it healthy and functioning. The heart in turn, needs a constant supply of oxygen-rich blood and nutrients to pump effectively. This is supplied by the coronary arteries which supply the heart muscle with oxygen and nutrients. When these 'highways' are clear and open, blood flows freely and smoothly both in the body and to the heart muscle. The heart too functions well. But when damage occurs to the coronary arteries which supply the heart muscle, and these pathways begin to narrow or become blocked, the heart struggles to get the blood it needs.

What Causes Damage to the Arteries

There are many factors that can damage the arteries, but one of the most significant is the buildup of a substance called *"Plaque"* in the walls of the arteries. The plaque is made up of various substances in the blood, including fat, cholesterol, calcium, and other materials. Over time, these substances can stick to and accumulate on the walls of the arteries, much like debris piling up on a road or pipes in our homes getting clogged with food waste or rust. This process is called *"Atherosclerosis"*, which is simply the hardening and narrowing of the arteries due to this buildup.

As the plaque accumulates on the artery walls, the space through which blood can flow becomes narrower. Think of it as a pipe that gets clogged over time. With less room for blood to flow, the heart has to work harder to pump blood, and sometimes the flow can be restricted so much that it causes serious problems.

The Impact of Narrowed or Blocked Arteries

As the arteries continue to narrow, the blood flow to the heart is reduced. This can lead to chest pain, commonly known as *"Angina"*, which occurs when the heart does not get enough oxygen during physical exertion or stress. Over time, if the blockage becomes severe, it can completely stop the flow of blood to certain parts of the heart, causing a heart attack.

Angina usually happens during moments when the heart is working harder, such as during exercise, stress, or even after a heavy meal. This is because the heart needs more oxygen during these activities, but if the arteries are too narrow, they cannot deliver enough blood to meet the excess demand. While angina can be alarming, it is often a signal that something is wrong with the blood flow to the heart, and it should never be ignored. It is the body's way of warning that the heart is struggling to get enough oxygen.

Silent Coronary Artery Disease
The Hidden Danger

Even though CAD is a serious condition, it often develops gradually over many years. Most people may not experience any symptoms in the early stages, which is why it is often referred to as a *silent* condition initially. However, if left untreated, CAD can lead to major complications, including heart attack and heart failure (when the heart cannot pump blood efficiently) or sudden *Cardiac Arrest* (when the heart suddenly stops beating).

In some cases, people can have Coronary Artery Disease (**CAD**) without experiencing any noticeable symptoms. This is known as *Silent CAD*. In silent CAD, the arteries may be narrowed, but the person does not feel any chest pain or other obvious warning signs. While silent CAD might seem less concerning because there are no symptoms, it is actually very dangerous. Because the person is unaware of the problem, they are at risk of having a heart attack without any prior warning. Thus for some people, the first sign of CAD may be the heart attack itself.

Silent CAD must be distinguished from *Silent Heart Attack*. The latter means heart attack occurring without symptoms and will be discussed later in detail.

Sudden Cardiac Arrest Risk
The Most Severe Complication

In the most severe cases, CAD can lead to *Sudden Cardiac Arrest* (**SCA**). Sudden cardiac arrest occurs when the heart suddenly stops beating. This is different from a heart attack, although the two are often related. A heart attack damages the heart muscle, but cardiac arrest affects the heart's electrical system, causing it to stop beating altogether suddenly.

When the heart stops beating, blood flow to the brain and other vital organs stops as well, and the person quickly loses consciousness. Without immediate medical intervention, sudden cardiac arrest is fatal. Emergency treatments, such as *Cardiopulmonary Resuscitation* (**CPR**) and *Defibrillation* (using an electric shock to restart the heart), are essential for survival. [See Chapter 24 on *Cardiac Arrest and Cardiopulmonary Resuscitation*].

Coronary Artery Disease

It is important to understand that CAD is a chronic condition, meaning it develops and progresses over time. It is not something that happens overnight. The damage caused by plaque buildup can begin as early as the 20s or 30s, but the symptoms may not appear until much later in life. This gradual progression makes it crucial to focus on prevention and early detection.

While CAD cannot be completely reversed, it can be managed effectively and its progression checked with lifestyle changes and, in some cases, medications or medical procedures. By understanding the causes and symptoms of CAD, individuals can take steps to reduce their risk and improve their heart health over the long term.

How the Heart Works and Why It Needs a Constant Blood Supply

As we have mentioned the heart is one of the most important organs in the human body. It is a muscular organ, roughly the size of your fist, and its main job is to pump blood throughout the body. This pumping action ensures that every cell receives the oxygen and nutrients it needs to function. On an average day, the heart beats around 100,000 times, sending blood to every corner of the body. But for the heart to keep doing this vital job, it needs its own supply of oxygen and nutrients. [See Chapter 3 on *Heart & the Circulatory System*].

The Heart's Need for Oxygen and Nutrients

Just like any other muscle in the body, the heart needs energy to work. This energy comes from oxygen and nutrients carried in the blood. Although the heart pumps blood to the entire body, it also requires a dedicated blood supply for itself. This supply comes from the '*Coronary Arteries*', which are small blood vessels that specifically feed the heart muscle. [See Chapter 2 on *Heart & the Circulatory System*].

Without a continuous supply of oxygen and nutrients, the heart muscle would struggle to pump blood effectively. If the blood flow to the heart is reduced or blocked, the affected parts of the heart muscle can become weak or, in more serious cases, begin to die. This can lead to dangerous complications, including heart attacks. In other words, for the heart to keep the rest of the body alive, it must first keep itself nourished.

How the Coronary Circulation Works

The coronary arteries keep the heart nourished. These arteries wrap around the heart, arising from its top like a 'crown'. Hence the name – *'Corona'* (Latin) means 'crown' or 'king'. These arteries ensure that oxygen-rich blood is delivered to every part of the heart muscle. These arteries are the heart's personal delivery system for oxygen and nutrients.

When everything is working well, this system keeps the heart beating steadily, ensuring it has enough energy to continue pumping blood throughout the body. But if something disrupts this system—such as a blockage in one of these arteries—the heart can quickly run into trouble. Without enough oxygen, parts of the heart muscle may stop working properly, leading to chest pain commonly known as *angina* or more serious issues like heart attacks. If the blood supply is cut off completely for too long, parts of the heart muscle can die, which can permanently weaken the heart.

Why the Heart's Blood Supply Is Vital for Other Organs

The heart plays a central role in keeping other organs in the body healthy. When the heart is strong and working well, it pumps oxygen-rich blood to vital organs like the brain, lungs, liver and kidneys. This keeps these organs functioning properly, allowing them to do their jobs, such as helping us breathe, filtering waste from the blood, and keeping our brain alert.

But when the heart does not get enough blood, it cannot pump blood as efficiently to the rest of the body. As a result, other organs begin to suffer. For example, the brain may not get enough oxygen, leading to dizziness, confusion, or even loss of consciousness in severe cases. The lungs may struggle to get the oxygen they need, which can make breathing difficult. The kidneys, which filter waste from our blood, may start to fail, causing harmful substances to build up in the body.

This is why maintaining a healthy blood flow to the heart is so crucial—not only for the heart itself but for the overall health of the body. This is why regular check-ups and monitoring for heart disease risk factors, like high blood pressure, high cholesterol, and diabetes, are so important. Even if a person feels perfectly fine, silent CAD could be developing, and early detection is key to preventing a heart attack.

In summary, the heart is the engine that keeps the entire body running. It needs a constant supply of oxygen and nutrients to function properly, and this is delivered through the coronary arteries. Without this supply, the heart muscle can weaken, leading to serious complications that can affect not just the heart but all the vital organs that depend on it. Taking care of our heart is essential for maintaining overall health, as it plays a vital role in keeping every part of our body working smoothly.

Key Takeaways

- *CAD is a condition where the arteries supplying blood to the heart become narrowed or blocked, often leading to heart attacks.*
- *Arteries are essential for delivering oxygen-rich blood and nutrients to the heart. When these arteries become damaged or blocked, the heart's blood supply is compromised, leading to potential health risks.*
- *CAD primarily develops due to atherosclerosis, where plaque (a mix of fat, cholesterol, and other substances) builds up inside the artery walls, narrowing them and restricting blood flow.*
- *Restricted blood flow can cause chest pain (angina) and, in severe cases, lead to heart attacks. Angina is a warning signal that the heart is struggling to get enough oxygen.*
- *CAD can be "Silent", (asymptomatic) meaning individuals may not experience noticeable symptoms until they suffer a heart attack, making regular check-ups vital for early detection.*
- *In the most critical cases, CAD can lead to sudden cardiac arrest, a life-threatening condition where the heart stops beating, and immediate medical intervention is necessary.*
- *CAD is a long-term, progressive condition that develops over many years. Prevention and early detection are key to managing its progression.*

- *The heart's blood supply is crucial for the health of all vital organs, and compromised blood flow can negatively impact the brain, lungs, kidneys, and other systems.*

Chapter 5 EPIDEMIOLOGY

Heart attacks, or Myocardial Infarctions, are one of the leading causes of death worldwide. Understanding how common they are, who they affect, and why their prevalence has increased over the years is essential for public health awareness This chapter explores the global statistics, regional differences, and how lifestyle changes have impacted the occurrence of heart attacks, both positively and negatively.

Prevalence and Incidence

Before we dive into the numbers, it is important to understand two key terms: *Prevalence* and *Incidence*. To understand the scope of heart attack or *Myocardial Infarction* (**MI**), it is imperative to distinguish between these two key epidemiological terms:

Prevalence: *This refers to the **total number** of people currently diagnosed with heart attack in a population at a given time.*

Incidence: *This refers to the number of **new cases** of heart attacks diagnosed over a specific period, typically one year.*

Both measures help us understand how widespread heart attacks are globally and how they are affecting populations over time.

Heart attacks are a major cause of death worldwide. According to the World Health Organization (**WHO**), *Cardiovascular Diseases* (**CVD**)—which include heart attacks—accounted for 17.9 million deaths in 2019, making them the leading cause of death globally. Of these deaths, 85% were due to heart attack and stroke. Heart attacks alone affect millions of people each year, and without timely medical intervention, they can be fatal. However, heart attacks are not only a global health issue; they also carry significant personal and societal burdens, leading to long-term health problems for survivors.

Global Burden

Heart attacks do not discriminate—they affect people from all regions of the world, regardless of socioeconomic status. However, there are key trends and differences in how heart attacks impact various countries.

In high-income countries, such as the United States, United Kingdom, and Australia, heart attacks are common, largely due to unhealthy lifestyle choices like poor diets, smoking, and lack of physical activity. However, improved healthcare and public health campaigns have started to lower heart attack rates in these nations. In the United States, heart disease, including heart attacks, is the number one cause of death, claiming around 697,000 lives annually. Every 40 seconds, someone in the U.S. suffers a heart attack. This makes it a public health crisis, costing not only lives but also impacting families and society at large.

Heart disease is the leading cause of death for men, women, and people of most racial and ethnic groups in the United States. It has been reported that in 2022, 702,880 people died from heart disease. That is the equivalent of 1 in every 5 deaths being due to heart attack. It is estimated that approximately one person dies every 33 seconds from cardiovascular disease. Heart disease cost about $252.2 billion from 2019 to 2020. This includes the cost of health care services, medicines, and lost productivity due to death.

Some of the projections and statistics published by the *American Heart Association* reveal the extent of the problem.

- *"Between 2000 and 2011, researchers found the national heart-related mortality rate declined at an average of 3.7 percent per year, while stroke mortality declined at 4.5 percent per year".*
- *"By 2035, nearly half of the U.S. population will have some form of cardiovascular disease."*
- *"At age 24, your risk for CVD is just 20 percent. By age 45, your chances more than double to 50 percent. Ninety percent of individuals over the age of 80 have some form of CVD."*
- *"In 2016, CVD cost America $555 billion. By 2035, the cost will skyrocket to $1.1 trillion."*
- *"In the next two decades, black Americans will have the highest rates of cardiovascular disease."*

In Europe, heart attacks also present a significant health challenge. Countries like the United Kingdom, Germany, and France report high numbers of heart attacks annually. For example, in the UK alone, about 100,000 hospital admissions occur each year due to heart attacks, which translates to roughly one heart attack every five minutes.

In low- and middle-income countries, such as India, China, and parts of Africa, heart attack rates are on the rise. This increase is driven by urbanization and economic development, which have introduced more sedentary lifestyles, increased consumption of processed foods, and greater stress levels.

In India, the situation is similarly alarming. Heart disease has become the leading cause of mortality in the country, with an estimated 2.1 million people (21 lakh) dying from heart-related conditions each year. Sedentary lifestyles, changes in diet, and increased stress levels are some of the contributing factors that have made heart attacks more common, even among younger individuals in urban areas.

China, the world's most populous country, has also seen a sharp rise in heart disease-related deaths, including heart attacks. Over the past few decades, rapid economic development has led to lifestyle changes that have increased the prevalence of risk factors like smoking, poor diet, and lack of physical activity. A total of 5.09 million CVD deaths were estimated in China in 2019. Of these, currently, more than 1 million people in China die from heart attacks each year.

These statistics are not just numbers—they represent real people, families, and communities affected by the devastating consequences of heart disease. They highlight the need for increased awareness, early detection, and better prevention strategies to reduce the global burden of heart attacks.

It is important to note that heart attacks are likely underreported in some regions, particularly in low-resource settings. In countries where healthcare access is limited, many heart attacks may go unrecognized or misdiagnosed due to a lack of diagnostic tools or trained medical personnel. As a result, the true global burden of heart attacks may be even higher than what is reported.

The prevalence of coronary artery disease (CAD) in the United States is around 4.6% of adults but varies by several factors. About 20.5 million U.S. adults have coronary artery disease, making it the most common type of heart disease in the United States.

Coronary heart disease killed 371,506 people in 2022 in the US. About 1 in 20 adults aged 20 and older have CAD (about 5%). Statistics report that in 2022, about 1 out of every 5 deaths from cardiovascular diseases (CVDs) was among adults younger than 65 years old.

In the United States, someone has a heart attack every 40 seconds. Every year, about 805,000 people in the United States have a heart attack. Of these, 605,000 are a first heart attack, and 200,000 happen to be people who have already had a heart attack.

The prevalence of CAD in Indians living in India is reported as 21.4% for diabetics and 11% for nondiabetics. In the rural parts of country, the prevalence of CAD is reported to be nearly half that in the urban population. In one major study, the overall prevalence of CAD among adults based on the clinical and ECG criteria was estimated as 9.7% and 2.7% in the urban and rural populations, respectively. In India in 2022, 32,457 people were reported to have died from heart attacks, which is a 12.5% increase from 2021. Still these figures could be an underestimate as many cases may go unreported. This revelation adds to the overall surge in sudden deaths, which reached a concerning 56,450 in 2022, marking a 10.1% increase from the previous year's figure of 50,739.

In China, out of a total of about 330 million people with cardiovascular disease (CVD) there are an estimated 11.39 million people with coronary artery disease (CAD). Cardiovascular disease is the leading cause of death in China, accounting for 46.74% of deaths in rural areas and 44.26% of deaths in urban areas in 2019.

Regional Variations in Heart Attack Incidence

High-Income Countries: In developed countries like the United States, Canada, and Western Europe, heart attack rates have historically been high due to factors such as high-fat diets, smoking, and stress. However, due to successful public health campaigns, better medical care, and increased awareness of heart health, heart attack rates in these countries have started to decline in recent decades.

Low- and Middle-Income Countries: The developing countries, particularly in South Asia, Africa, and parts of Latin America, are now experiencing a sharp increase in heart attack cases. As urbanization spreads, more people adopt sedentary lifestyles, consume processed foods, and face increased levels of stress. Unfortunately, these regions also tend to have limited access to healthcare, leading to worse outcomes for heart attack victims.

Eastern Europe and Russia: Heart attack rates in parts of Eastern Europe and Russia remain high, due in part to higher smoking rates, excessive alcohol consumption, and poor access to preventive healthcare. Public health campaigns and improved healthcare infrastructure are needed to address the persistent high rates in these regions.

Between 1960 and 1990, however, the death rate due to coronary artery disease dropped by 30% in the European union testifying to the improvement in care and the steps taken towards public education and prevention.

Differences Across Age Groups

Heart Attacks in Older Adults: Heart attacks are most common in older adults. People over the age of 65 are at a significantly higher risk because of age-related changes in the heart and blood vessels. Over time, arteries tend to stiffen, and plaque buildup (known as *atherosclerosis*) increases, making older individuals more vulnerable to blockages that cause heart attacks.

Rising Incidence in Younger Populations: While heart attacks were traditionally seen as a condition affecting older adults, there has been a worrying rise in cases among younger people, particularly men under 50. This increase is linked to lifestyle factors such as obesity, diabetes, smoking, and drug use (especially substances like cocaine). Sedentary behavior and poor dietary habits also contribute to this alarming trend.

Differences Between Genders

Men and Heart Attacks: Men are generally more prone to heart attacks at younger ages than women. This is because men tend to develop coronary artery disease earlier in life. Risk factors such as smoking, high cholesterol, and high blood pressure are more prevalent in men, further increasing their susceptibility to heart attacks in their 40s and 50s.

<u>Women and Heart Attacks:</u>   While men are more likely to have heart attacks earlier in life, women are at increased risk of heart attacks later, particularly after menopause. Before menopause, women have higher levels of estrogen, a hormone that helps keep arteries flexible. However, after menopause, estrogen levels drop, and women become more vulnerable to heart disease. Women often experience different heart attack symptoms than men—such as fatigue or back pain—which can delay diagnosis and treatment. As a result, women have higher mortality rates following a heart attack.

<u>Gender Disparities in Treatment</u>:   Studies suggest that women are less likely than men to receive aggressive treatment for heart attacks, such as surgery or medications, which contributes to their higher mortality rates. Closing this gender gap in treatment could save countless lives.

Public Health Impact Of Heart Attack

The public health impact of heart attacks extends beyond the individuals affected. It places an immense strain on healthcare systems around the world. In countries with advanced healthcare infrastructure, like the U.S. and Europe, heart attacks lead to billions of dollars in medical expenses each year. This includes emergency room visits, hospitalizations, surgeries and cardiac procedures (such as bypass surgeries and angioplasty), and long-term care for heart disease patients.

For example, in the U.S., heart disease costs the healthcare system about $229 billion annually. This includes direct medical costs as well as indirect costs from lost productivity and premature death. When people suffer a heart attack, they often need months or even years of follow-up care and rehabilitation, putting a long-term burden on healthcare providers and insurers.

In developing countries, where healthcare systems are often less equipped to deal with chronic conditions, the impact is even more severe. Heart attacks not only lead to high treatment costs but also result in lost productivity, particularly when younger individuals are affected. The economic toll is particularly significant when breadwinners or key workers are unable to continue their jobs due to the long-term effects of a heart attack.

Moreover, heart attacks contribute to the growing global health disparities. Access to quality healthcare and preventive measures varies widely between countries and even within regions. Rural areas in many countries may not have the same access to emergency care as urban centers, leading to higher mortality rates in those regions. This highlights the need for global initiatives to address heart disease through education, better healthcare access, and prevention programs.

Why Heart Attacks Are More Common Today

Several factors have contributed to the rise in heart attacks in recent decades.

Changes in Diet

<u>Increased Caloric Intake</u>: Modern diets, particularly in urbanized areas, are often high in calories, leading to weight gain and obesity. Obesity is a major risk factor for heart disease, as it raises the likelihood of developing conditions such as high blood pressure and diabetes.

<u>Saturated Fats and Trans Fats</u>: The widespread use of processed foods, which are high in saturated and trans fats, has played a significant role in increasing heart disease rates. These unhealthy fats contribute to the buildup of plaque in the arteries, which can lead to blockages and heart attacks. Although trans fats have been reduced or banned in many countries, their long-term impact on heart health continues to be felt.

<u>Sedentary Lifestyles</u>: Modern technology has made many aspects of life easier, but it has also contributed to a more sedentary lifestyle. Desk jobs, longer commutes, and screen-based entertainment have all contributed to a reduction in physical activity. Regular exercise is essential for maintaining a healthy heart, and without it, people are more likely to develop high blood pressure, obesity, and heart disease.

<u>Increase in Smoking</u>: The 20th century saw a dramatic rise in smoking rates, particularly among men. Smoking is a major risk factor for heart disease, as it damages the lining of the arteries and encourages plaque buildup. Although smoking rates have declined in many countries thanks to anti-smoking campaigns, it remains a significant risk factor in regions where tobacco use is still prevalent.

<u>Higher Stress Levels</u>: As modern life becomes faster paced and more demanding, stress levels have increased. Chronic stress raises blood pressure and leads

to unhealthy coping mechanisms such as overeating, smoking, or excessive alcohol consumption. Stress also contributes to poor sleep, which further increases the risk of heart disease and heart attacks.

Rise of Diabetes and Obesity: The global rise in obesity and diabetes has become a major public health concern. Both conditions significantly increase the risk of heart attacks. High blood sugar levels, a hallmark of diabetes, damage blood vessels and impair the heart's ability to function properly. Obesity, on the other hand, puts additional strain on the heart, contributing to high blood pressure and cholesterol levels. As more people develop these conditions, heart attack rates continue to climb.

Lifestyle Changes
Positive Changes in Lifestyle

Public Health Campaigns: Over the past few decades, many governments and health organizations have launched successful public health campaigns aimed at reducing heart disease risk. Anti-smoking initiatives, exercise promotion, and campaigns encouraging healthier diets have all contributed to a decline in heart attack rates, particularly in high-income countries.

Better Awareness and Screening: People are now more aware of the risks associated with high blood pressure, high cholesterol, and diabetes. Routine screenings for these conditions have become more common, allowing for earlier intervention. The use of medications like *Statins* (to lower cholesterol) and blood pressure-lowering drugs has helped millions reduce their heart attack risk.

Improvements in Emergency Care: Advances in medical care, especially in Prehospital care and

Emergency heart attack treatment, have saved countless lives. Modern treatments, including clot-busting drugs and procedures to reopen blocked arteries, have greatly improved survival rates.

Negative Lifestyle Changes

Processed Foods and Sugary Beverages: The global availability of processed foods and sugary drinks has skyrocketed, leading to increased rates of obesity, diabetes, and heart disease. Western-style fast food has had particularly harmful effects in regions like Asia and the Middle East, where heart attack rates have risen dramatically.

Decrease in Physical Activity: While advances in technology have made life more convenient, they have also reduced the need for physical activity. Many people now lead sedentary lives, which contributes to heart disease.

Thus, CAD is the leading cause of heart attacks and a major global health issue accounting for significant morbidity and mortality worldwide, particularly in developed nations. CAD incidence increases with age, affecting more men than women, though this gap narrows post-menopause. Risk factors include hypertension, high cholesterol, smoking, diabetes, and a sedentary lifestyle. The prevalence of CAD is rising due to aging populations, unhealthy diets, and increasing rates of obesity and diabetes.

Key Takeaways

- *Heart attacks are a leading cause of death globally, with millions of cases occurring each year, particularly in developed nations and rapidly urbanizing regions.*

- *Incidence rates are rising in low- and middle-income countries due to lifestyle changes, including unhealthy diets, increased stress, and reduced physical activity.*
- *Developed countries have seen a decline in heart attack rates due to improved healthcare, public health campaigns, and awareness of risk factors like smoking and high cholesterol.*
- *Heart attack incidence increases with age and is more common in men, though the gender gap narrows after menopause.*
- *Younger populations are now experiencing rising heart attack rates due to obesity, smoking, and drug use.*
- *Women often face higher mortality rates from heart attacks, in part due to delayed diagnosis and differences in symptoms from men.*

Chapter 6 ANGINA PECTORIS

Angina pectoris, commonly known as 'angina', is a type of chest pain or discomfort that occurs when the heart does not get enough oxygen-rich blood. It often serves as a warning sign of an underlying heart condition, particularly coronary artery disease (CAD), where the arteries become narrowed or blocked. Understanding angina is crucial because it helps patients recognize symptoms early, allowing for timely medical intervention and lifestyle adjustments to prevent more serious heart problems, such as a heart attack.

This chapter focuses on educating the public about the differences between stable and unstable angina, their symptoms, triggers, and when to seek immediate medical attention. By learning how to manage angina and recognizing its role as the heart's "alarm bell," patients can take important steps to protect their heart health and improve their quality of life.

Angina pectoris, commonly referred to as angina, is a type of chest pain or discomfort caused by reduced blood flow (*ischemia*) to the heart muscle. The term "*Angina Pectoris*" is derived from the Latin words '*angere*', which means 'to choke', and '*pectus*', which means 'chest'. The literal translation of the term is "the choking of the chest". While it may sound alarming, it is important to know that angina is not a disease in itself but rather a symptom of an underlying heart condition. Understanding angina is crucial because it serves as a warning sign that the heart is not getting the blood and oxygen it needs, particularly during times when it is working harder.

What is Angina?

Angina often occurs when the heart does not receive enough oxygen-rich blood because the blood vessels that supply the heart—called *coronary arteries*—become narrowed or blocked. The reduced blood flow limits the heart's ability to work efficiently, especially when it needs to pump harder, such as during physical activity or emotional stress. As a result, the heart struggles to keep up, leading to chest pain or discomfort.

Link to Coronary Artery Disease

In most cases, angina is closely linked to *Coronary Artery Disease* (**CAD**). CAD occurs when the arteries that supply blood to the heart become narrowed due to the buildup of fatty deposits called *plaque*. This condition restricts blood flow and makes it harder for the heart to get the oxygen it needs, particularly during times of exertion or stress. Thus, when the heart's demand for oxygen rises, but the narrowed arteries cannot supply enough blood, the person may experience angina.

People often describe angina as a sensation of pressure, tightness, or heaviness in the chest. Some say it feels like someone is squeezing their chest. The pain can also spread to other parts of the body, such as the arms, shoulders, neck, jaw, or back. Angina is usually brief, lasting only a few minutes, but it can be very uncomfortable. Often the angina is relieved when the factor which caused it is removed. Thus when the exercising person rests or the stressed person calms down, the angina disappears.

Angina is not a heart attack but a warning sign. Although angina can feel like a heart attack, it is not the same thing. Angina does not cause permanent damage to the heart muscle. However, it is an important signal that something is wrong with the blood flow to the heart. Angina should not be ignored, as it indicates an increased risk of more serious heart problems, such as a heart attack.

There are two main types of angina: *Stable* and *Unstable*. Understanding the difference between the two is important because one is predictable and generally manageable, while the other is unpredictable, more dangerous and requires immediate medical attention.

Stable Angina

Stable angina occurs when the heart has to work harder than normal, such as during physical exertion, emotional stress, or even after eating a large meal. It follows a predictable pattern, meaning that people who experience stable angina can often anticipate when it will occur and what activities trigger it. For example, climbing a flight of stairs, walking two blocks, shoveling snow in winter or walking uphill may cause chest pain.

The common triggers for stable angina include:

- <u>Physical exertion</u>: Activities like walking, running, or carrying heavy objects can increase the heart's demand for oxygen and precipitate an attack of angina. Climbing stairs is a common situation when susceptible persons develop angina.

- <u>Emotional stress</u>: Strong emotions, such as anxiety, stress or anger, can cause the heart to work harder and precipitate an attack of angina.

- <u>Eating a heavy meal</u>: After eating a large meal, the heart may need more oxygen to help with digestion and angina may occur. After a large meal, the body diverts more blood towards the digestive system, thus depriving the already affected heart of the much needed oxygen.

The pain or discomfort from stable angina typically goes away after a few minutes of rest or with medication. Nitroglycerin (*Glyceryl Trinitrate*) tablet is a common medication given *sublingually* (under the tongue) to relieve angina symptoms. It works by relaxing (*dilating*) blood vessels, allowing more blood to flow to the heart. In addition, learning to manage stress and avoid known triggers can help reduce the frequency of angina episodes.

Stable angina thus has a predictable nature, and the patient often knows which activities or circumstances precipitate an attack of angina. Most patients learn to avoid such situations which can provoke angina. While stable angina can be uncomfortable, it is generally not life-threatening if managed properly. It is a sign that there is an ongoing problem with the heart's blood supply, but it can often be controlled with lifestyle changes and medications. However, it is still important to monitor stable angina closely, as it can progress if left untreated. **[Fig 6.1]**.

Unstable Angina

Unstable angina also called (*Acute Coronary Syndrome* or **ACS)** is more serious than stable angina. It does not follow a predictable pattern and can occur even when a person is at rest. This makes it more dangerous, as the lack of blood flow to the heart can happen without warning, and the pain may be more severe and last longer.

With unstable angina, symptoms may occur at rest, become more frequent, severe, or prolonged than the usual pattern of angina and change from the usual pattern of angina. It may or may not respond to rest or medications immediately. *"Stuttering Angina"* is one which comes and goes without a predictable pattern and can happen prior to a heart attack.

Unstable angina suggests that the heart's blood supply is becoming more restricted. This is a sign that the condition is getting worse. Because the blood flow to the heart is more severely reduced, unstable angina is a more urgent and serious condition. It is considered a medical emergency because it often signals that a heart attack could happen soon. If a person experiences chest pain that does not go away or gets worse, it is important to seek immediate medical attention, as it could be a sign of an impending heart attack.

How Angina Warns Us About Potential Heart Problems

Angina pectoris is not just a sign of discomfort—it is an important early warning system that can signal potential heart problems. By understanding how angina works, we can take steps to protect our hearts before more serious conditions, like a heart attack or a sudden cardiac arrest, occur.

Angina pectoris is the heart's anguished cry, a deep, suffocating ache that yearns desperately for the life-giving flow of blood, as if caught in a fleeting grasp of sorrow – to put it figuratively.

Angina acts like the heart's alarm bell. It occurs when the heart is not receiving enough oxygen-rich blood, usually because the coronary arteries that supply the heart are narrowed or blocked. The pain or discomfort associated with angina is the heart's way of telling us that something is wrong. When the heart needs more oxygen, like during exercise or stress, and the blood flow is restricted, the heart signals this imbalance through the symptoms of angina.

One of the most important roles of angina is its ability to alert us before a more serious problem arises. It gives people an opportunity to address heart issues before they lead to a heart attack, which causes permanent damage to the heart muscle. Recognizing and responding to the symptoms of angina can save lives. If you notice these symptoms early, you can seek medical help, make lifestyle changes, or start treatments that can reduce the strain on your heart and lower the risk of a heart attack.

Angina is often connected to other health issues beyond the heart itself. High blood pressure (*Hypertension*), high cholesterol (fatty substances in the blood), and diabetes can all contribute to the occurrence of angina as these diseases can cause atherosclerosis of the coronary arteries. Treating these underlying conditions is critical. By managing high blood pressure, reducing cholesterol levels, and controlling blood sugar, people can reduce chances of developing angina and improving their overall heart health.

When Angina Becomes Dangerous

Angina can progress from a manageable condition to a more dangerous one. While stable angina follows a predictable pattern, unstable angina is more unpredictable and poses a much higher risk. A person with stable angina may find that his angina has become unstable if it occurs frequently, the angina changes its nature, and the pain lasts for longer than normal or it is felt in other places like the jaw or arms or if it occurs at rest. Hence it is called *Acute Coronary Syndrome* (**ACS**) – a transition between stable angina and a heart attack. This form of angina that often presages a heart attack is a medical emergency that requires immediate attention. Regular medical checkups are important to monitor the progression of angina and adjust treatment as needed to keep the heart healthy.

Symptoms of Angina

Recognizing the symptoms of angina is key to understanding what is happening in your heart. The discomfort felt during an angina episode often follows a particular pattern, but the sensations can vary from person to person. Recapitulating the symptoms of angina, it is most commonly felt as:

- A tightness or pressure in the chest, as if something heavy is pressing down on it.

- A squeezing sensation in the center of the chest that can spread (*radiate*) to other areas of the body, such as the arms, shoulders, neck, jaw, or back (between the shoulder blades).

- A burning feeling or a sense of fullness in the chest that some people might mistake for indigestion or heartburn.

These sensations are usually brief, lasting a few minutes, but they can be alarming.

Other Symptoms Beyond the Chest

While chest discomfort is the most recognized symptom of angina, not everyone experiences it in the same way. Other symptoms can include:

- Discomfort in the arms, neck, jaw, or stomach alone without pain in the chest - pain can sometimes be felt in areas other than the chest.

- Some people feel like they cannot catch their breath, especially during physical activity and feel excessively short of breath.

- Feeling sweaty or having cool, moist skin can accompany angina.

- Some may feel light-headed or queasy during an angina episode.

For those with stable angina, the symptoms usually last just a few minutes and improve with rest or medication. However, unstable angina can last longer and does not respond as easily to rest or medication. Physical exertion, emotional stress and large meals are often the common triggers for angina to develop.

> *Desmond, a 40-year-old smoker, a clerk in a government concern, first felt a tightness in his chest one evening while walking briskly to catch the bus. Dismissing it as indigestion or stress, he ignored the discomfort. However, the sensation returned a few days later as he climbed a flight of stairs—this time sharper and accompanied by shortness of breath. Concerned, Desmond visited a cardiologist. After a thorough evaluation, including an ECG treadmill stress test and Coronary Angiography, he was diagnosed with Stable Angina Pectoris, caused by a narrowed coronary artery reducing blood flow during exertion.*
>
> *But as the blockage in his coronary artery was not very critical, his doctor prescribed medications, including nitrates and beta-blockers, and recommended lifestyle changes such as quitting smoking, eating a heart-healthy diet, and regular, moderate exercise. Over time, Desmond's symptoms eased, and he regained control of his health, avoiding further complications. He continued to be on regular follow up.*

How to Recognize the Difference Between Angina and a Heart Attack

It is important to distinguish between the symptoms of angina and a heart attack, as the two can feel similar but have different levels of severity.

Angina pain typically lasts for a short period (3-5 minutes), happens during physical activity or stress, and usually improves quickly with rest or medication whereas a heart attack pain lasts longer than 10 minutes, does not go away with rest, and is often more intense. It may be accompanied by severe shortness of breath, weakness, or a sense of impending doom.

The discomfort and chest pain caused by angina can be frightening, especially if it is unexpected and occurs for the first time. Many people experience anxiety or fear during an angina episode, as the symptoms can be alarming. The worry that it could be a heart attack can increase stress and make the episode feel more overwhelming. Learning to manage this fear is important in handling angina episodes calmly.

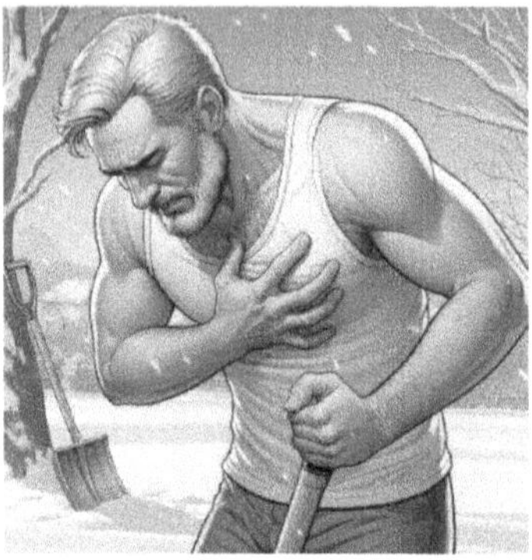

Fig 6.1 An attack of angina working in cold weather

Factors That Worsen Angina

Certain factors can make angina worse or trigger episodes more frequently. Being aware of these can help in managing the condition better.

Cold Weather: Cold temperatures can cause blood vessels to *constrict* (narrow), making it harder for blood to flow to the heart. This can trigger angina episodes, especially during physical activity in cold weather like shoveling snow.

> *Sam, a 50-year-old man, experienced sudden chest pain while arguing with his boss at the office. The discomfort lasted about five minutes and eased when he returned to his desk to rest. He brushed it off, but later that night, after dinner, while relaxing and watching TV, the same pain resurfaced, this time lasting nearly 20 minutes. He felt mild palpitations but attributed the discomfort to indigestion, avoiding telling his wife to prevent worrying her.*
>
> *Hours later, Sam was jolted awake in the middle of the night with a choking sensation, severe breathlessness, and a cold sweat. Alarmed, he woke his wife, and they rushed to the emergency room. The resident doctor quickly diagnosed stuttering Unstable Angina after an abnormal ECG, and a cardiologist was called in. Sam was given medications to relieve his pain, and an emergency coronary angiogram revealed a critical narrowing in a major coronary artery. Immediate angioplasty was performed, restoring blood flow. His pain subsided, and the post-angioplasty ECG returned to normal. Sam was prescribed medications and lifestyle changes and advised to attend regular checkups. The prompt intervention of the medical team had helped him narrowly avoid a heart attack.*

<u>Large Meals</u>: Digesting a heavy meal requires more blood flow to the digestive system, which can take away from the heart's blood supply and trigger angina.

<u>Smoking or Secondhand Smoke</u>: Smoking damages blood vessels and reduces the oxygen level in the blood, making angina worse. Chronically being exposed to secondhand smoke can also have a similar harmful effect. Also, severe air pollution as has been seen in some countries during winter (smog) can trigger attacks of angina in susceptible persons.

Management of Angina Pectoris

Angina pectoris, characterized by chest pain due to myocardial ischemia, requires a multi-faceted approach for effective management. Key strategies include lifestyle modifications, pharmacological interventions, and, in severe cases, invasive procedures.

General Measures

<u>Lifestyle Modifications</u>: Smoking cessation, weight management, regular physical activity, and dietary changes (low-fat, low salt) are foundational for reducing cardiovascular risk.

<u>Risk Factor Control</u>: Managing risk factors like hypertension, high blood cholesterol, and diabetes is crucial to reducing angina frequency and improving long-term outcomes.

Pharmacological Therapy

<u>Nitrates</u>: Nitroglycerin, used as quick dissolving tablets under the tongue (*sublingual*) or as long-acting

forms, provides rapid relief by dilating coronary arteries and reducing myocardial oxygen demand.

<u>Beta-blockers</u>: These agents (e.g., *Metoprolol, Carvedilol*) reduce heart rate and the work of the heart muscle thus lowering the oxygen requirement of the heart and thereby and preventing angina episodes.

<u>Calcium Channel Blockers</u> (**CCBs**): Drugs like *Amlodipine, Verapamil* or *Diltiazem* help by *dilating* (widening) the coronary vessels and reducing work of the heart, making them effective for those intolerant to beta-blockers.

<u>Antiplatelet Agents</u>: Low-dose *Aspirin* or *Clopidogrel* is commonly prescribed to prevent clots in the coronary arteries and reduce the risk of myocardial infarction. These are blood thinners that reduce the risk of blood clotting which is the hallmark of a heart attack.

<u>Ranolazine</u>: This newer medication works by reducing sodium and calcium overload in the heart cells, providing symptom relief, particularly in difficult cases.

Non-Pharmacological Treatments

<u>Percutaneous Coronary Intervention</u> (**PCI**): Involves *Angioplasty* and *Stenting* to restore blood flow in stenotic coronary arteries, offering relief from angina in patients with significant coronary artery disease.

<u>Coronary Artery Bypass Grafting</u> (**CABG**): A surgical option for patients with severe or multiple blockages, CABG improves blood flow by bypassing the occluded arteries.

Emerging Therapies

Enhanced External Counter Pulsation (**EECP**): A non-invasive treatment that improves blood flow and reduces angina symptoms in patients who are not candidates for surgery.

Gene Therapy and Stem Cell Therapy: These experimental therapies are being explored for promoting formation of new blood vessels in the heart and repairing the damaged heart tissue, offering hope for the future treatment of difficult to treat angina.

In summary, the management of angina involves a combination of lifestyle interventions, medications, and, when needed, surgical approaches to improve symptoms and prevent further cardiac events. More regarding these will be discussed in Chapter 15 on *Hospital Management of Heart Attack*.

Preventive Measures

Living with angina does not mean you cannot take steps to improve your heart health and reduce the frequency of symptoms. Some lifestyle changes that can help include:

Quitting smoking: Smoking is one of the biggest risk factors for heart disease. Quitting can significantly improve blood flow and reduce the risk of angina and heart attacks.

Eating a heart-healthy diet: A diet rich in fruits, vegetables, whole grains, and lean proteins can help lower cholesterol and blood pressure, reducing the risk of angina.

Managing stress: Stress can trigger angina, so learning relaxation techniques or engaging in calming activities can help. Also, avoiding emotional outburst and being overly emotional can help.

Regular physical activity: Exercise strengthens the heart and improves blood circulation. However, it is important to consult a doctor about safe exercise routines if you have angina. [See Chapter 20 on *Prevention of Heart Attack*].

Importance of Seeking Medical Advice

If you experience angina symptoms, it is essential to seek medical attention. A doctor can help diagnose the underlying cause, whether it is coronary artery disease or another heart condition. Early diagnosis and treatment can prevent more serious problems, like heart attacks, and improve your quality of life.

Angina serves as a critical reminder that the heart is under strain. By recognizing the signs and addressing the underlying causes, we can protect our hearts and improve our overall health. The management of stable and unstable angina will be dealt with in the chapters on management.

In conclusion, angina is a warning sign that the heart's blood supply is inadequate, often due to narrowed coronary arteries. While stable angina can be controlled, unstable angina is a serious condition that requires immediate attention. Recognizing the symptoms and understanding the differences between stable and unstable angina can help individuals take timely action to protect their heart health.

Key Takeaways

- *Angina pectoris is a symptom of reduced blood flow to the heart, often caused by narrowed coronary arteries.*
- *Angina is not a disease in itself but a symptom of underlying heart conditions, most commonly coronary artery disease (CAD).*
- *Stable angina occurs predictably during physical exertion or stress, and symptoms typically improve with rest or medication like nitroglycerin.*
- *Unstable angina is more dangerous, can happen at rest, and signals worsening heart conditions, requiring immediate medical attention.*
- *Symptoms of angina include chest pain or discomfort that may radiate to the arms, neck, jaw, back, or shoulders, often described as tightness, pressure, or squeezing.*
- *Angina is distinct from a heart attack, though the sensations may feel similar; heart attacks cause permanent heart damage, while angina does not.*
- *Managing underlying conditions like high blood pressure, high cholesterol, and diabetes is critical in reducing angina episodes and improving heart health.*
- *Cold weather, large meals, stress, and smoking can worsen angina by increasing strain on the heart or reducing oxygen flow.*
- *Early recognition and treatment of angina can prevent more serious heart problems, such as heart attacks, and improve long-term outcomes.*

Chapter 7 HEART ATTACK (MYOCARDIAL INFARCTION)

A heart attack, also known as a Myocardial Infarction (MI), is a life-threatening condition that occurs when the blood supply to part of the heart muscle is blocked. This blockage, usually caused by a buildup of plaque in the coronary arteries, deprives the heart of oxygen, leading to damage or death of the heart tissue.

This chapter describes the causes, symptoms, and urgent care needed for a heart attack, or Myocardial Infarction (MI). It explains how blockages in the coronary arteries prevent oxygen from reaching the heart muscle, leading to damage or tissue death. Recognizing key symptoms such as chest pain, shortness of breath, and fatigue, as well as understanding the differences between a heart attack and angina, is essential for seeking immediate medical help. The chapter emphasizes the importance of early detection and timely treatment to minimize heart damage and improve recovery.

A heart attack, also known as a *Myocardial Infarction* (**MI**), is a serious medical condition where the blood flow to a part of the heart is severely reduced or completely blocked. This blockage prevents the heart from receiving the oxygen it needs to function, and if untreated, it can cause permanent damage to the heart muscle. Understanding what happens during a heart attack and why it occurs is essential for recognizing its symptoms and seeking timely medical care.

What is a Heart Attack?

A heart attack occurs when the flow of blood to a section of the heart muscle is suddenly reduced or stopped altogether. The heart, like all muscles, relies on a steady supply of oxygen and nutrients to work properly. This oxygen-rich blood is delivered to the heart through the coronary arteries, which act as vital highways supplying the heart muscle.

In most cases, the problem arises due to a buildup of substances like fat, cholesterol, and other materials (*Plaque*) within the arteries. Over time, these substances can harden, narrow, or even rupture, forming a blood clot that blocks the artery. When the artery is totally blocked, oxygen cannot reach the part of the heart that it normally supplies. Without enough oxygen, the heart muscle begins to suffer, and this lack of oxygen leads to damage or death of the heart tissue, known as a heart attack.

Why is it Called "Myocardial Infarction"?

The medical term for a heart attack is *"Myocardial Infarction"*. *'Myo'* refers to muscle, *'Cardia'* refers to the heart and '*Infarction*' means the death of tissue due to a lack of blood supply.

So, <u>*Myocardial Infarction literally means the death of the heart muscle due to an insufficient blood supply*</u>. This explanation is important because it reminds us that the heart, although a strong and hardworking organ, is still a muscle that needs constant oxygen to keep working properly. If that oxygen supply is interrupted, the heart muscle becomes damaged, and over time, this damage can seriously affect the heart's ability to pump blood throughout the body.

What Happens to the Heart Muscle During a Heart Attack?

The heart's main job is to pump oxygen-rich blood to the rest of the body, but it also needs a continuous supply of blood to keep working. When a heart attack occurs, the blood supply to part of the heart muscle is suddenly cut off, depriving that section of the heart of oxygen. This lack of oxygen causes the affected area of the heart muscle to weaken and stop functioning properly. If the oxygen supply is not restored quickly, the damage begins to set in and becomes permanent.

One of the critical aspects of a heart attack is how quickly it is treated. The longer the heart muscle goes without oxygen, the more severe the damage becomes. Doctors often say, "*time is muscle*," meaning the faster medical treatment is received, the more heart muscle can be saved. For example, treatments such as medication to dissolve clots or surgical procedures to restore blood flow (like *Angioplasty*, which opens blocked arteries) can minimize damage if administered quickly.

The left ventricle is the part of the heart most commonly affected by a myocardial infarction (heart attack) due to its high oxygen demand, resulting from its crucial role in pumping blood throughout the body. While myocardial infarction primarily impacts the left ventricle, damage can sometimes extend to the right ventricle or even the atria.

If the blockage lasts too long, however, the heart muscle in the affected area begins to die. Once this damage occurs, it becomes permanent, and the heart loses part of its ability to pump effectively. This is why it is critical to treat a heart attack as an emergency and seek medical help immediately.

The heart's ability to pump blood depends on the strength of its muscle. When part of the heart muscle is damaged or destroyed during a heart attack, the heart can no longer work as efficiently. This reduced function can lead to long-term conditions, such as heart failure, where the heart is unable to pump enough blood to meet the body's needs. The severity of the heart failure depends on how much of the heart muscle was damaged during the heart attack.

After a heart attack, the body tries to repair the damaged heart muscle, but instead of forming new healthy heart muscle, it creates scar tissue. The heart muscle cells, unlike the cells in the liver or skin cannot regenerate to form new heart muscle cells. While scar tissue helps 'patch up' the damaged heart, this scar does not have the same strength or flexibility as healthy heart muscle. Scar tissue does not contract or contribute to the heart's pumping action, which can further reduce the heart's ability to function properly. Over time, this can lead to complications, including irregular heartbeats (*Arrhythmias*) or heart failure.

Signs and Symptoms of a Heart Attack

Heart attacks often present with several recognizable symptoms, but it is crucial to remember that not everyone experiences the same warning signs. Understanding these symptoms can save lives. *Symptoms* are what the patient complains of, and *Signs* are what the doctor finds on examination.

Chest Pain or Discomfort

The most common symptom of a heart attack is chest pain or discomfort. Many people describe it as a feeling of intense pressure, squeezing, or fullness in the center of the chest, like a heavy weight pressing down. Even though the symptoms are akin to those of angina, unlike angina, this discomfort typically lasts more than a few minutes, and it may transiently disappear briefly but then return. The pain is often persistent and does not improve with rest, which distinguishes it from angina and other less serious conditions.

The chest pain is the hallmark of a heart attack, but it does not always stay confined to the chest. The discomfort may *radiate* (spread) to other areas, such as the arms (especially the left arm), the neck or jaw, the shoulders, or the back. This happens because the nerves that carry pain signals from the heart also connect to these areas of the body, causing the pain to spread.

Shortness of Breath

Many people experience shortness of breath during a heart attack, even when they are not physically active. This occurs because the heart struggles to pump blood efficiently when its oxygen supply is cut off. As a result, the body, including the lungs, does not receive enough oxygen, leading to difficulty in breathing. Shortness of breath can also occur due to a complication of heart attack called *Acute Pulmonary Edema* where fluid accumulates inside the lungs. [See Chapter 16 on *Complications of Heart Attack*].

Other Symptoms

In addition to chest pain and shortness of breath, a heart attack may trigger other symptoms that may seem unrelated at first but are crucial warning signs.

Sweating: Breaking out in a cold sweat is common as the body reacts to the stress of the heart attack. Patients may find that their clothes are often drenched with sweat.

Nausea and vomiting: Some people feel sick to their stomach or vomit during a heart attack. This may be mistakenly attributed to indigestion by the patient.

Lightheadedness or dizziness: Reduced blood flow to the brain can cause a person to feel dizzy or faint during a heart attack. The decrease in blood pressure during a heart attack may also cause the patient to feel faint.

Fatigue: Feeling excessively tired or exhausted, especially for women, is a common but often overlooked symptom. This is also attributed to the inability of the heart to pump enough blood or to a lowered blood pressure.

Silent Heart Attack

In some cases, heart attacks occur without the classic symptom of chest pain, particularly in older adults, women, or people with diabetes. These are called *Silent Heart Attacks* or *Silent Myocardial Infarction* (**SMI**). Instead of intense chest pain, they may experience more subtle symptoms, such as fatigue, mild discomfort, or shortness of breath, which can easily be mistaken for something less serious. Silent heart attacks can be just as dangerous, hence it is important to pay attention to these less obvious signs also.

Differences Between Angina and Heart Attack

While angina and heart attacks share similar symptoms, they are not the same. Angina is a warning sign that the heart is not getting enough oxygen-rich blood, but it is usually less severe than a heart attack. Angina has already been discussed in the previous chapter.

While the symptoms of angina and a heart attack can be similar, there are important differences. They are:

- Angina does not cause permanent damage to the heart muscle. A heart attack, however, leads to muscle damage due to the prolonged lack of oxygen.
- Angina pain often goes away with rest or medication, but heart attack pain persists and worsens over time.

- Angina typically lasts for a few minutes and improves with rest or removal of the triggering factor, while a heart attack lasts longer and does not get better with rest.
- Angina occurs when the heart temporarily does not get enough oxygen. A heart attack happens when blood flow is completely blocked, causing muscle damage.

However, it is important to recognize when angina might be signaling an impending heart attack. If angina pain becomes more frequent, lasts longer, or occurs while at rest, it could indicate that a heart attack is about to happen. This condition is *Unstable Angina* and requires immediate medical attention.

The Importance of Early Detection

Recognizing the early signs of a heart attack is important to save lives. Many people delay seeking help because they do not realize they are having a heart attack, especially if their symptoms are mild or mistaken for indigestion. Early detection is crucial because the longer you wait, the more damage is done to the heart. If you or someone you know experiences the symptoms of a heart attack, it is important to act fast and seek medical help quickly.

First Aid During a Heart Attack

If you suspect that someone is having a heart attack, take the following steps immediately:

<u>Call emergency services:</u> Time is critical in reducing heart damage, so do not hesitate to call for medical help.

Chew an aspirin (if not allergic): Aspirin can help thin the blood, improving blood flow to the heart. If a clot has formed, aspirin prevents the clot from growing in size. However, aspirin should be given only if the person is not allergic to aspirin and emergency services have been contacted. The person should not have any stomach problems like peptic ulcer and should not have been advised to avoid aspirin by his doctor. More details are discussed in Chapter 13 on *Prehospital Management of Heart Attack*.

The management is dealt with in detail in Chapters 14 and 15. Prevention has been dealt with in detail in Chapter 20.

In summary, a heart attack is a serious event caused by the blockage of blood flow to the heart muscle. Untreated, this lack of oxygen causes the heart muscle to become damaged or die. Knowing the signs and symptoms of a heart attack, how it differs from angina, and the steps one can take during an emergency can make all the difference.

Key Takeaways

- *A heart attack, or Myocardial Infarction (MI), occurs when blood flow to part of the heart is blocked, depriving the heart muscle of oxygen and causing damage or death to the tissue.*
- *The term "Myocardial Infarction" means the death of heart muscle tissue due to insufficient blood supply.*
- *Heart attacks are primarily caused by a blockage in the coronary arteries, often due to plaque*

- *buildup (Atherosclerosis), which can lead to a blood clot.*
- *Symptoms include chest pain, shortness of breath, sweating, nausea, dizziness, and fatigue. These can vary, especially in women and older adults, who may experience more subtle signs.*
- *Timely treatment is critical—early intervention, such as dissolving clots or restoring blood flow through procedures like angioplasty, can minimize damage to the heart muscle.*
- *Silent heart attacks (Silent Myocardial Infarction) can occur without the typical severe chest pain and can be just as dangerous, making it important to recognize less obvious symptoms like mild discomfort or fatigue.*
- *Heart muscle damage from a heart attack is permanent, and scar tissue that forms in place of the damaged muscle reduces the heart's ability to pump effectively, leading to potential complications like heart failure or arrhythmias.*
- *Heart attack symptoms differ from angina, as angina pain usually subsides with rest or medication, while heart attack pain persists and worsens without treatment.*
- *Early detection and seeking immediate medical care can save heart muscle and reduce long-term damage. Acting quickly during a heart attack is vital to improving survival and recovery outcomes.*

Chapter 8 CAUSES OF HEART ATTACK

Heart attacks, also known as myocardial infarctions, occur when the heart is suddenly deprived of oxygen-rich blood, leading to damage to the heart muscle. This is most commonly caused by blockages in the coronary arteries due to a buildup of plaque, a process known as Atherosclerosis. When a plaque ruptures, it can lead to the formation of a blood clot, which can completely block blood flow, triggering a heart attack. Other causes, such as coronary artery spasms or genetic factors, can also increase heart attack risk.

Educating the public on the causes of heart attacks is crucial for prevention. Understanding how lifestyle choices, such as diet, exercise, and smoking, affect heart health can empower individuals to take steps to reduce their risk.

A heart attack, also known as a *Myocardial Infarction* (**MI**), occurs when the heart suddenly loses its supply of oxygen-rich blood. Let us explore the main causes of a heart attack, focusing on the role of blockages in the coronary arteries and the sudden formation of blood clots.

The Coronary Arteries

The coronary arteries are the essential blood vessels that supply the heart muscle with the oxygen and nutrients it needs to function. Like any other muscle in the body, the heart requires a constant flow of oxygenated blood to keep it healthy and working efficiently. These arteries wrap around the outside of the heart, ensuring every part of the muscle receives the blood it needs. [See Chapter 3 on *Heart & Circulatory System*].

How Blockages Form

The most common cause of a heart attack is a blockage in one or more of these coronary arteries. Over time, these blockages form as a result of a gradual buildup of plaques inside the artery walls. A *Plaque* is a sticky substance made up of fat, cholesterol, and other materials like calcium and proteins. The process - the hardening and narrowing of the arteries due to build up of plaque inside the arteries, is called *Atherosclerosis*.

As the plaque forms on the inner walls of the coronary arteries, it narrows the space through which blood can flow. This reduces the amount of oxygen-rich blood that can reach the heart muscle. For most people, this process happens slowly over the course of years or even decades. The person, when resting, may not notice any symptoms. However, during physical exertion or stress, the heart needs more blood, and the narrowed arteries cannot meet that demand, leading to chest pain which is known as *angina*. When a clot blocks the artery completely, it results in a heart attack.

Vulnerability of Plaques

Some plaques are *'stable'* and remain attached to the artery wall without causing immediate problems. However, other plaques are more *'vulnerable'* and can be easily damaged and hence *rupture* (break open). Plaque rupture is often triggered by factors like high blood pressure or inflammation in the artery walls. When a plaque ruptures, it exposes its contents to the bloodstream, setting off a chain reaction that can lead to a heart attack.

Although atherosclerosis develops gradually, the impact of a heart attack can be sudden and severe. When a plaque ruptures, it can quickly lead to the formation of a blood clot on top of it, which is the immediate cause of most heart attacks. This sudden event can block the artery completely, cutting off the supply of oxygen to the heart muscle causing a heart attack.

Formation of a Blood Clot

When a plaque inside the coronary artery ruptures, the body responds as it would to any injury—it tries to heal the damage. The body sends *platelets* (tiny blood cells that help in clotting) to the site of the rupture. Platelets are constantly circulating in the blood. These platelets stick together initially, and form a blood clot, which normally helps to stop bleeding. However, in the case of a ruptured plaque, the clot forms inside an already narrowed artery. Instead of helping, the clot thus becomes a blockage in the artery, cutting off the flow of blood to that section of the heart completely.

Thus, when the blood clot completely blocks the artery, oxygen-rich blood and nutrients can no longer reach the heart muscle. Within minutes, the cells in that part of the heart get injured and begin to die as they are starved of oxygen. This is what happens during a heart attack. The heart muscle depends on a continuous supply of oxygen, and when it is cut off, damage begins rapidly. This is why heart attacks are medical emergencies that require immediate treatment.

Heart Damage from Blood Clots

The severity of the heart attack depends on two factors - the size of the blood clot and how long the artery remains blocked. The longer the blockage lasts, the more heart muscle is damaged. If the blood flow is not restored quickly, the damage can become permanent, leading to weakened heart function or even heart failure (where the heart cannot pump blood as effectively as it should). This is why it is so important to get medical help as soon as heart attack symptoms appear.

While plaque rupture is the most common cause of blood clot formation, rarely blood clots form in coronary arteries without any plaque rupture. Certain conditions can make the blood more likely to clot, such as specific blood disorders or illnesses that increase clotting tendencies. In these cases, a heart attack can occur even if the person does not have severe atherosclerosis.

Symptoms of Heart Attack

When a heart attack occurs, the symptoms we associate with it—such as chest pain, shortness of breath, and nausea—are directly caused by the heart muscle being deprived of oxygen. The blood clot blocking the artery is what triggers these symptoms. As the heart struggles to function without its normal supply of oxygen, it sends out distress signals in the form of pain and discomfort.

Coronary Artery Spasm

Coronary artery spasms are an uncommon but a serious cause of heart attacks. *A spasm is the sudden contraction of a muscle such as a cramp.* Unlike the typical cause of heart attacks—blockages from plaque or clots, these spasms occur when the muscles in the walls of the coronary arteries suddenly tighten and narrow. This tightening can drastically reduce or even completely block the flow of blood to the heart. When blood flow stops, the heart does not get the oxygen it needs, which can lead to a heart attack.

There are a few causes of coronary spasms which we will see in brief:

- Smoking is a major factor that can lead to coronary artery spasms. The chemicals in cigarettes irritate the inner lining of the arteries, making them more likely to spasm or tighten suddenly.
- Certain drugs, particularly cocaine and amphetamine, can trigger these spasms. Cocaine overstimulates the nervous system, causing

intense tightening (*constriction*) of the arteries even in people who do not have plaque buildup. This makes drug use especially dangerous for the heart.
- Exposure to extremely cold temperatures can cause coronary artery spasms, which is why more heart attacks tend to occur in colder months. The cold constricts the arteries, making spasms more likely.
- High levels of emotional stress or anxiety can trigger a surge of stress hormones like adrenaline. Adrenaline makes the arteries *constrict* (tighten), which increases the likelihood of a coronary spasm. Stress also affects the overall health of the heart, contributing to long-term heart problems.

While a coronary artery spasm is often temporary, it can cause serious harm if it lasts long enough to significantly reduce or block blood flow to the heart. The lack of oxygen can injure the heart muscle, and if this happens repeatedly, it can lead to a chronic form of heart disease. Repeated spasms increase the risk of more severe heart problems over time, even though each episode may only last a few minutes.

Diagnosing coronary artery spasms can be tricky because they do not always show up on standard heart tests, like *Angiograms* (imaging tests that look for blockages). These spasms tend to happen unexpectedly and might not be present during testing. Doctors may instead monitor a person's heart rhythm or blood pressure over time or use special tests to provoke a spasm in a controlled setting to see how the arteries respond. This can help determine if coronary artery spasms are the reason for the heart problems.

> Sara, a 35-year-old mother of four young children, had been dealing with frequent, intense episodes of chest pain. These episodes seemed to come on during times of emotional stress, but each time she went to her doctor, her ECG results were normal. Her physician couldn't identify the exact cause of her pain and decided to refer her to a cardiologist.
>
> The cardiologist performed a coronary angiogram, which also appeared normal. To investigate further, he conducted a special test to provoke a response in her coronary arteries. During this test, Sara's right coronary artery suddenly went into spasm, causing the chest pain she had been describing. The spasm was quickly relieved with sublingual nitroglycerin, confirming the diagnosis of coronary artery spasm.
>
> With this understanding, Sara was prescribed medications to prevent further spasms. She was also advised to see a counselor for help in managing stress, a known trigger for her condition. Thanks to this combined treatment, Sara's chest pain episodes stopped, allowing her to focus on her family and daily life without the constant worry of unpredictable pain.

Genetic (Inherited) Factors
Family History of Heart Disease

Genetics plays a significant role in heart disease. If you have a family history of heart disease, especially if close relatives (like parents or siblings) had heart attacks at an early age, your own risk of CAD is higher. This increased risk is due to inherited traits that can make you more likely to develop conditions that lead to heart attacks, such as high cholesterol, high blood pressure (*hypertension*), or diabetes.

Inherited Conditions That Increase Risk

1. <u>Familial Hypercholesterolemia</u>: One of the most common inherited conditions that raises the risk of heart attacks is called familial hypercholesterolemia. This condition causes very high cholesterol levels, even from a young age. Cholesterol is a fatty substance that can build up in the arteries, leading to plaque formation. This plaque formed due to the high blood cholesterol can clog the arteries, making it harder for blood to flow to the heart. People with familial hypercholesterolemia often experience heart attacks much earlier in life, sometimes before they reach the age of 50.

2. <u>Genetic Predisposition to High Blood Pressure</u> (*Hypertension*): High blood pressure is another key risk factor for heart attacks. Some people are genetically predisposed to develop high blood pressure, meaning they inherit a tendency to have elevated blood pressure levels, even if they lead a healthy lifestyle. High blood pressure puts extra strain on the arteries, weakening them over time. This makes it easier for plaque to build up, which can lead to heart attacks.

3. <u>Diabetes and Insulin Resistance</u>: Genetics also influences the risk of developing diabetes, a condition where the body does not use insulin properly, leading to high blood sugar levels. Over time, high blood sugar can damage blood vessels and make it more likely for plaque to build up, increasing the risk of blockages that cause heart attacks. People with diabetes have double the risk of heart attacks compared to those without the condition.

Thanks to advances in medical science, genetic testing is now available to help people identify whether they carry specific genes that increase their risk of heart disease. If you have a family history of heart attacks, genetic testing can be a useful tool for early prevention. By knowing your inherited risk, you can take proactive steps to protect your heart, by adopting preventive

> *Mahesh and Suresh, 27-year-old twins, had both pursued individual business ventures after losing their father to a heart attack at the age of 47. One day, Mahesh was rushed to the emergency department with intense chest pain and severely low blood pressure, indicative of a massive heart attack complicated by Cardiogenic Shock. Despite the medical team's relentless efforts, Mahesh passed away within six hours.*
>
> *Following his brother's tragic death, Suresh underwent comprehensive testing, revealing high cholesterol levels of 360 mg/dL. Diagnosed with Familial Hypercholesterolemia, he was prescribed high-dose atorvastatin and scheduled for regular follow-ups. His Treadmill Stress Test, however, did not show any evidence of coronary artery disease. Initially diligent, Suresh kept his appointments for two years but eventually stopped attending follow ups.*
>
> *Five years later, one evening Suresh was brought in to the emergency room, this time with severe chest pain and an Anterior Wall Myocardial Infarction. Emergency angioplasty saved his life, though he admitted to discontinuing his medication and skipping follow-ups. His cholesterol had soared to 630 mg/dL, and he had gained significant weight. After a stern warning from his cardiologist, Suresh was discharged a week later and enrolled in a cardiac rehabilitation program to help manage his condition and prevent future incidents.*

measures. Early prevention can make a significant difference in reducing your risk of a heart attack.

Gene-Environment Interaction

It is important to remember that while genetics plays a role in the risk of heart disease, it is not the only factor. Lifestyle choices such as diet, physical activity, smoking, and how one handles stress have a huge impact on whether or not a person will actually develop heart disease. For example, even if one is genetically predisposed to high blood pressure, leading a healthy lifestyle can help keep it under control and lower the risk of a heart attack.

Although some causes of heart disease, like genetics and coronary artery spasms, may be out of one's control, many risk factors are preventable. By leading a healthy lifestyle, an individual can significantly reduce the risk of heart attacks, even if one has a genetic predisposition or a family history of heart disease. Small but consistent habits like eating a balanced diet, exercising regularly, not smoking, and managing stress can make a big difference in keeping your heart healthy.

Regardless of the cause—whether it is due to blocked arteries, a blood clot, coronary artery spasms, or genetics—the end result is the same—the heart muscle suffers when it does not get enough blood. Quick treatment is vital to restore blood flow and minimize damage to the heart. Understanding the different causes of heart attacks helps in recognizing risks early and taking steps to prevent serious outcomes.

By taking proactive steps and seeking medical advice when necessary, one can protect the heart and reduce the likelihood of a heart attack, even if certain risk factors are beyond one's control. Prevention is the key to heart health.

Key Takeaways

- *A heart attack occurs when the heart is deprived of oxygen-rich blood, usually due to blockages in the coronary arteries, leading to damage to the heart muscle.*
- *Blockages in coronary arteries are commonly caused by atherosclerosis, the gradual buildup of plaque inside artery walls, narrowing them over time.*
- *Plaque ruptures can trigger blood clot formation, which may completely block the artery and cause a heart attack by cutting off the oxygen supply to part of the heart muscle.*
- *The severity of heart damage from a heart attack depends on the size of the clot and how long the artery remains blocked.*
- *In rare cases, coronary artery spasms—sudden tightening of the artery walls due to factors like smoking, drugs, cold temperatures, or stress—can also lead to a heart attack without plaque buildup.*
- *Genetics can increase the risk of heart attacks, especially through conditions like familial hypercholesterolemia, inherited high blood pressure, or diabetes, which contribute to artery blockages.*
- *While some causes, like genetics or coronary artery spasms, are uncontrollable, many risk factors, such as poor diet, lack of exercise,*

smoking, and stress, can be managed to lower the risk of heart attacks.
- *Rapid medical intervention is critical during a heart attack to restore blood flow and minimize heart damage. Understanding the causes can aid in prevention and timely treatment.*

Chapter 9 RISK FACTORS FOR HEART ATTACK

Heart attacks remain a leading cause of death worldwide but understanding the risk factors can empower individuals to take control of their heart health. This chapter will explore both modifiable and non-modifiable risk factors for heart attacks, highlighting how lifestyle choices such as diet, exercise, smoking, and stress play a key role in causing a heart attack. While factors like age, genetics, and family history cannot be changed, awareness can help individuals recognize early signs, make healthier decisions, and manage existing conditions like high blood pressure, diabetes, and high cholesterol. Patient education is critical in encouraging small but effective lifestyle changes that can significantly reduce heart attack risks and lead to a longer, healthier life.

Heart attacks are one of the leading causes of death worldwide, but understanding the factors that increase the risk is important to make informed choices to protect one's heart. Some of the major and lifestyle-related risk factors for heart attacks are discussed below, focusing on how everyday habits and health conditions can influence heart health.

Modifiable and Non-Modifiable Risk Factors

Heart attacks do not happen without warning. There are some risk factors that predispose an individual to a heart attack. Some of these risk factors can be changed by altering our lifestyle or by appropriate treatment whereas others cannot be changed.

By understanding the risk factors—both those that can be controlled, like diet and exercise, and those that cannot, like family history or age—one can take action to protect the heart. Based on the changes that one can make to reduce the risk factors, they have been classified into two categories namely, *Modifiable Risk Factors* and *Non-modifiable Risk Factors*.

The Modifiable risk factors are those that individuals can change or be controlled through lifestyle choices or medical intervention. These include Smoking, High blood pressure (*hypertension*), High cholesterol levels, Diabetes, Obesity, Physical inactivity, Unhealthy diet, Excessive alcohol consumption and Chronic stress. Small, consistent lifestyle changes can have a big impact on reducing the chances of a heart attack and keeping the heart strong and healthy for years to come, by changing or controlling these factors.

On the contrary, the Non-modifiable risk factors are those factors that cannot be changed. These include

Age, Gender, Family history, Genetic predispositions and Ethnicity.

Managing modifiable risk factors through healthy lifestyle changes can significantly lower heart attack risk, even for those with other non-modifiable risk factors.

Modifiable Risk Factors

Some of the modifiable risk factors are very important and hence are called the *Major Risk Factors*. They are discussed below.

High Blood Pressure (*Hypertension*)

High blood pressure, or *hypertension*, occurs when the force of blood pushing against the walls of the arteries is consistently too high. Blood pressure naturally rises and falls throughout the day, but when it stays elevated for long periods, it becomes dangerous.

When the heart contracts, the blood pressure rises; this is called the *Systolic Blood Pressure* (**SBP**). When the heart relaxes, the blood pressure falls to a lower level; this is called the *Diastolic Blood Pressure* (**DBP**). The blood pressure is expressed in *millimeters of the mercury* (**mmHg**). The normal SBP is between 120-130 mmHg and the normal DBP is 80 mmHg or lower. The blood pressure reading is thus expressed as 130/80 mmHg. Elevations of blood pressure above these levels are considered to be high.

Over time, the increased pressure can damage the artery walls, making them more prone to the buildup of plaque. This buildup can cause blockages that reduce or stop the flow of blood to the heart, leading to a heart attack.

When blood pressure is high, the heart must work harder to pump blood throughout the body. This extra strain can weaken the heart muscle. Initially, the heart muscle becomes thickened (*Hypertrophy*) but over time it makes the heart muscle less efficient. Additionally, high blood pressure damages the inner lining of arteries (*Endothelium*), making it easier for harmful substances like cholesterol and fat to stick to the walls, eventually forming *plaques* and blockages. These blockages restrict blood flow to the heart, which increases the risk of a heart attack.

High Cholesterol

Cholesterol is a fatty substance that is essential for building cells and producing certain important hormones. However, too much cholesterol in the blood can lead to the buildup of plaque in the arteries, increasing the risk of heart attacks.

LDL (*Low-Density Lipoprotein*): Known as "*bad cholesterol*," LDL is responsible for plaque formation in the arteries, making them narrower and harder.

HDL (*High-Density Lipoprotein*): Often called the "*good cholesterol*," HDL helps remove the deposited cholesterol from the arteries and transport it to the liver, where it can be processed and eliminated from the body. It thus scavenges the cholesterol deposited in arterial walls.

The normal blood level for Total Cholesterol is considered to be less than 200 mg/dL, LDL cholesterol should be less than 100 mg/dL, and HDL cholesterol should be at least 40 mg/dL for men and 50 mg/dL for women. Higher HDL levels are considered better.

When LDL cholesterol levels are high, cholesterol begins to accumulate in the arteries, leading to the formation of plaque. Over time, this plaque hardens and narrows the arteries, limiting the blood flow to the heart. If the plaque breaks, it can form a clot on top of it which blocks the artery, cutting off the flow of blood.

Below (**Table 9.1**) is a table with the normal ranges of various lipids in the blood of an adult. These ranges are generally accepted as indicators of *lipid* (fatty substances) levels in a healthy adult.

Lipid Type	Normal Range mg/dL	Normal Range (mmol/L)
Total Cholesterol	< 200	< 5.2
LDL Cholesterol	< 100	< 2.6
HDL Cholesterol	40 – 60	1.0 – 1.5
Triglycerides	< 150	< 1.7
Non-HDL Cholesterol	< 130	< 3.4

Table 9.1: Normal Ranges of Lipids

Values outside these ranges may indicate an increased risk of cardiovascular disease and may require medical attention and lifestyle changes.

Smoking

Smoking is one of the most significant preventable risk factors for heart attacks. The harmful chemicals in cigarette smoke damage the lining of the arteries, making it easier for fatty substances to build up and form blockages. Smoking also raises blood pressure and reduces the oxygen in the blood, forcing the heart to work harder to deliver oxygen throughout the body.

Cigarette smoke contains toxic chemicals that tend to make the blood thicker and more likely to form clots. These clots can block arteries, which can trigger a heart attack.

Even if one does not smoke, being exposed to second-hand smoke (inhaling the smoke released from someone else's cigarette) can increase one's risk of heart disease. It can damage the heart and blood vessels in much the same way as if the person were smoking himself.

Diabetes

Diabetes is a condition where the body either does not produce enough insulin (a hormone that helps regulate blood sugar) or cannot use insulin effectively. This leads to high levels of sugar (*glucose*) in the blood.

The normal Fasting Blood Glucose is below 100 mg/dL. If the blood taken two hours after food (*Postprandial*) shows a blood sugar level less than 140 mg/dL (7.8 mmol/L), it is considered normal.

If the blood sugar level 2 hours after food is between 140 and 199 mg/dL (7.8-11.0 mmol/L), it means that the person has *Prediabetes*, which is a warning sign for potential future diabetes and if the blood sugar level is 200 mg/dL (11.1 mmol/L) or higher, it indicates that the person has diabetes. [**Table 9.2**].

Hemoglobin A1c (**HbA1c**) is a blood test that measures the average amount of glucose, or blood sugar, in the blood over the past two to three months. It is also known as a *Glycated Hemoglobin* test.

High blood sugar from diabetes can damage blood vessels and the nerves that control the heart. It also increases the likelihood of plaque buildup in the arteries, which can restrict blood flow and trigger a heart attack. Diabetes is of two main types:

Result	Plasma Glucose (mg/dL)	Plasma Glucose (mmol/L)	HbA1C (%)	Diagnosis
Fasting Plasma Glucose	Less than 100	Less than 5.6	Below 5.7	Normal
Fasting Plasma Glucose	Between 100 – 125	Between 5.6 – 6.9	Between 5.7 – 6.4	Prediabetes
Fasting Plasma Glucose	Above 126	Above 7	Above 6.5	Diabetes mellitus

Table 9.2: Normal and Abnormal Values of Blood Sugar.

Type 1 diabetes is where the body does not *produce* insulin, so the blood sugar levels must be controlled with insulin injections.

Type 2 diabetes is where the body does not use insulin properly, leading to high blood sugar levels. Type 2 diabetes is more common and often linked to lifestyle factors such as diet and exercise.

Lifestyle-Related Factors

Lack of Exercise

Regular physical activity is one of the most effective ways to keep one's heart healthy. Exercise strengthens the heart, improves blood circulation, and lowers blood pressure. It also helps regulate body weight, blood sugar, and cholesterol levels, all of which are important for reducing the risk of heart attacks.

A sedentary lifestyle weakens the heart and reduces circulation, increasing the risk of high blood pressure, obesity, and poor cholesterol control. Over time, these factors contribute to the development of heart disease and heart attacks. Studies have shown that a lack of physical activity is linked to 7-12% of heart attack cases, making it a significant factor in heart health.

Even moderate physical activity, like walking briskly for 30 minutes a day, can lower an individual's risk of heart problems. Consistency is key—regular movement helps maintain heart health and prevent complications.

Unhealthy Diet

What one eats has a significant impact on one's heart health. Diets high in saturated fats, trans fats, cholesterol, and sodium (salt) can increase the risk of plaque buildup in the arteries, high blood pressure, and high cholesterol—all major contributors to heart attacks.

Some of the foods which should be avoided to reduce the risk of heart disease are:

- Processed foods which often contain high amounts of unhealthy fats and sodium, which raise blood pressure and cholesterol.

- Sugary drinks and snacks containing too much sugar can lead to weight gain and increase the risk of diabetes.

- Fried foods are typically high in trans fats, which raise the LDL ('bad') cholesterol levels.

Some of the Heart-healthy foods are eating more fruits, vegetables, whole grains, and lean proteins (such as fish and chicken) can improve heart health. Foods rich in fiber and omega-3 fatty acids, like nuts, seeds, and fatty fish, help reduce cholesterol and inflammation, which protects the heart.

Obesity

Carrying extra weight, especially around the abdomen, puts additional strain on the heart. It raises blood pressure, cholesterol, and blood sugar levels, creating a perfect storm of risk factors for heart attacks.

The fat that accumulates around the internal organs like liver, stomach, intestines and kidneys (*Visceral Fat*) is particularly dangerous. This type of fat produces chemicals that increase inflammation in the body, damaging the heart and arteries over time.

Small changes in one's lifestyle make a big difference. Even modest weight loss—5-10% of one's total body weight—can significantly improve heart health by lowering blood pressure, cholesterol, and blood sugar levels. These improvements can dramatically reduce the risk of a heart attack.

Other Important Modifiable Risk Factors

Let us now explore the roles of some more of modifiable risk factors like Stress, Alcohol, and Substance abuse in increasing heart attack risk. We will also look at non-modifiable risk factors like Family History and Aging, which, although unchangeable, can be managed with awareness and preventive steps.

Stress

Stress is an inevitable part of life, but when it becomes *chronic* (long-lasting), it can have a harmful effect on the heart. Chronic stress often leads to unhealthy habits such as overeating, smoking, or excessive drinking, all of which can contribute to heart disease. Even without these behaviors, stress itself can increase heart attack risk by raising blood pressure and promoting inflammation in the body. Stress has been found to contribute to about 3% of heart attacks.

When a person is stressed, the body activates a *"fight or flight"* response, releasing stress hormones like *Adrenaline*. This causes the heart to beat faster and the blood vessels to *constrict* (narrow), temporarily raising blood pressure. Over time, frequent or prolonged stress responses can damage the arteries, increasing the risk of heart attacks. Stress can also make it harder for the heart to function effectively, particularly in people who already have heart disease.

Managing stress is essential for heart health. Simple techniques like regular exercise, deep breathing, meditation, leisure time activities or spending quality time with friends and family can help reduce stress levels. Finding time to unwind can lower blood pressure and protect one's heart. The key is to incorporate relaxation practices into one's daily life to reduce the harmful effects of chronic stress on the heart. Getting 7 – 8 hours of sleep daily can also be an effective way to relieve stress.

Alcohol Consumption

Alcohol can have different effects on the heart depending on how much a person drinks. While some studies suggest that moderate alcohol consumption—such as one glass of wine a day—might have heart-protective effects, excessive drinking can be harmful. Drinking too much alcohol raises blood pressure, contributes to weight gain, increases cholesterol and triglyceride (another type of fat) levels, and can lead to irregular heartbeats, all of which raise the risk of heart disease.

Over time, heavy drinking can weaken the heart muscle, a condition called *Cardiomyopathy* (when the heart muscle becomes weak). This makes it harder for the heart to supply the body with enough oxygenated blood, leading to fatigue and potentially more serious conditions like heart failure. Drinking in moderation—if at all—is key to protecting heart health.

Substance Abuse

Substance abuse, especially the use of drugs like cocaine or methamphetamine, poses a serious risk to heart health. These stimulants cause an immediate and extreme rise in heart rate and blood pressure, which can trigger a heart attack even in people with no previous heart conditions. Cocaine, in particular, can cause coronary artery spasms (sudden tightening of the arteries), which can completely block blood flow to the heart.

Although marijuana is often viewed as less harmful than other drugs, smoking it can still strain the heart. It increases heart rate and blood pressure, putting extra pressure on the cardiovascular system. For people with pre-existing heart conditions or those at high risk, marijuana use can increase the chances of a heart attack or stroke. A recent study from the United States showed that the daily use of cannabis — predominately through smoking — was associated with a 25% increased likelihood of heart attack and a 42% increased likelihood of stroke when compared to non-use of the drug.

Lesser-Known Modifiable Risk Factors for Heart Attacks

Environmental factors, particularly air quality, play a significant role in cardiovascular health. Pollutants in the air, such as carbon monoxide, nitrogen dioxide, sulfur dioxide, and particulate matter, have been associated with increased heart attack risk. Short-term exposure to these pollutants can trigger inflammatory responses in the body, leading to a cascade of events that may culminate in a myocardial infarction. These pollutants not only stress the respiratory system but also place additional strain on the heart and circulatory system. Research has shown that even brief exposures to high levels of air pollution can elevate the risk of heart attacks and other acute cardiovascular events.

People working irregular hours, especially shift workers, are also at a higher risk of experiencing heart issues. Interestingly, research indicates a rise in heart attack cases immediately following the start of daylight saving time, likely due to the sudden shift in sleep patterns. These findings highlight the impact of lifestyle factors on heart health.

Non-Modifiable Risk Factors
Family History

Your family history refers to the health conditions that have affected your close relatives, such as your parents, siblings, or grandparents. If heart disease is common in your family, your own risk of developing heart problems is higher. This is because genetics play a role in determining how your body handles cholesterol, blood pressure, and how quickly your arteries might harden or become blocked.

Genetics can influence key factors like cholesterol levels, blood pressure, and how your body metabolizes fats. If you inherit certain genetic traits, you may be more prone to developing conditions like high blood pressure, high cholesterol, or diabetes, all of which increase the risk of heart attacks.

Being aware of your family's health history is a valuable tool in preventing heart disease. If you know that heart disease runs in your family, you can take proactive steps to reduce your own risk. Regular check-ups with your doctor, early lifestyle changes (like improving your diet or increasing exercise), and monitoring key health indicators such as blood pressure and cholesterol can help prevent or delay the onset of heart disease.

Age

As we age, the risk of heart disease increases. The arteries naturally become less flexible and more prone to narrowing due to age. Over time, these blockages can lead to heart attacks. This is partly due to changes in the body's ability to regulate cholesterol and blood pressure as well as the cumulative effects of lifestyle choices over the years.

The risk of heart disease begins to increase more noticeably as people get older. Men over the age of 45 and women over the age of 55 are at higher risk of having a heart attack.

Aging affects the heart in several ways. The heart muscle may weaken or stiffen, making it harder for the heart to pump blood effectively. Additionally, the arteries may lose some of their elasticity, which makes it easier for plaque to build up and harder for blood to flow freely. High blood pressure and diabetes, which become more common as people age, also contribute to the risk of heart disease.

While certain risk factors like family history and age cannot be changed, many other risk factors can be controlled through lifestyle choices. Taking charge of your health by managing these risk factors can significantly reduce the risk of heart attacks.

Key Takeaways

- *Heart attacks are one of the leading causes of death worldwide, but many risk factors can be managed through lifestyle changes.*
- *Risk factors for heart attacks fall into two categories: modifiable (e.g., smoking, high blood pressure, diet) and non-modifiable (e.g., age, genetics).*
- *High blood pressure, cholesterol levels, smoking, diabetes, obesity, and lack of exercise are major modifiable risk factors for heart attacks*
- *Smoking significantly raises heart attack risk by damaging artery walls and increasing blood clot formation.*
- *Managing diabetes and maintaining healthy cholesterol levels are critical for reducing plaque buildup in the arteries, which can lead to heart attacks.*
- *Lifestyle factors like regular exercise and a healthy diet rich in fiber, fruits, and lean proteins can lower the risk of heart disease.*
- *Chronic stress and excessive alcohol consumption also contribute to heart disease by raising blood pressure and weakening the heart.*
- *Age, family history, and genetic predispositions are non-modifiable risk factors, but awareness of these can help in taking preventive steps early.*

Chapter 10 PATHOPHYSIOLOGY OF HEART ATTACK

A heart attack, or myocardial infarction, happens when the heart muscle is starved of oxygen due to a blocked artery, leading to serious and potentially life-threatening damage. In this chapter, we explore the pathophysiology of heart attacks, breaking down how plaques buildup in the arteries, inflammation, and blood clots contribute to this condition. Understanding these processes is key for patients to recognize the importance of managing risk factors like high blood pressure, cholesterol, and smoking.

A heart attack, also known as a *Myocardial Infarction*, is a serious medical emergency that happens when the heart muscle is deprived of oxygen due to a blocked artery. Understanding how this occurs can help us better grasp why early treatment is so crucial in preventing permanent damage to the heart. Let us break down, in simple terms, how heart attacks develop—from the formation of blockages to the life-threatening damage they cause to the heart.

The term "*Pathophysiology*" refers to the <u>study of abnormal changes in body functions that are the causes, consequences, or concomitants of a disease processes</u>. Now, let us discuss the pathophysiology of how a heart attack begins and how it progresses.

The heart gets its blood supply through the *Coronary Arteries*, which are small vessels that wrap around the heart like tiny tubes. These arteries deliver oxygen-rich blood to the heart muscle, allowing it to pump blood throughout the rest of the body. However, if one of these arteries becomes clogged, the part of the heart that depends on that artery's blood supply is starved of oxygen. This is what causes a heart attack.

A heart attack starts when blood flow to a section of the heart is suddenly blocked. When the blood supply to the heart is interrupted, the affected part of the heart does not get the oxygen it needs to function. Without oxygen, the heart muscle begins to suffer damage, and the longer the blockage lasts, the worse the damage becomes. If the blockage is not cleared quickly, the heart muscle can die, which can lead to serious complications or death.

During a heart attack, time is of the essence. The longer the blockage remains, the more damage is done to the heart muscle. Every minute without oxygen leads to the death of more heart muscle cells. That is why it is essential to get immediate medical help if you or someone else experiences symptoms of a heart attack. Physicians often quote "*Time is Muscle*", meaning that the more time is lost in getting treatment for the patient, the more of the heart muscle is at risk of being damaged. Quick treatment can reopen the blocked artery and restore blood flow to the heart, minimizing damage.

We have seen that plaques which are the sticky, fatty deposits that form on the inner walls of arteries consist of cholesterol, fat, calcium, and other substances found in the blood. Over time, they enlarge and narrow the arteries, making it harder for blood to flow freely. This gradual buildup is the starting point for most heart attacks.

The Atherosclerotic Plaque

Let us see how the atherosclerotic plaque develops and grows.

The process begins when the inner walls (*Endothelium*) of the arteries are damaged. A plaque develops from a thin layer of cells which accumulate in the endothelium of the artery. The first visible sign of atherosclerosis is called a *Fatty Streak*. It is a yellow patch or streak of dead white blood cells that form at the site of damage to the inner lining of the artery. These white blood cells have accumulated fat inside them and appear foamy. They are called the "*Foam cells*".

Soon, more dead white blood cells and other debris build up at the site, turning the fatty streak into a larger raised '*plaque*'. On the surface of the plaque is formed a thick cover of fiber-tissue which is called a *Fibrous Cap*. This increases gradually and the plaque grows in size causing a partial block in the artery. The fibrous cap may be thin and may be vulnerable to damage and rupture. When it is thicker, the chances of rupture are less.

Sometimes, the thin fibrous cap that covers the plaque may break open, or the endothelial cells around the plaque wear away (*eroded*), allowing a blood clot to form on top of the plaque. This clot may totally block blood flow, which can lead to a heart attack. The *Plaque* is made up of cholesterol, fatty substances, cellular waste products, calcium, and a protein called *fibrin*. [**Fig 10.1**]

What causes the fibrous cap to be damaged or rupture?

A sudden damage or rupture of the thin fibrous cap of the plaque can be caused by factors like high blood pressure, smoking, or high levels of cholesterol in the blood. Plaque buildup does not happen overnight—it is a slow and relentless process. This process is known as *Atherosclerosis*. It can take years or even decades for enough plaque to build up to cause a problem. During this time, the artery gradually narrows, and blood has a harder time flowing through. This can lead to symptoms like chest pain (*Angina*) when the heart is not getting enough blood during physical activity or stress.

Stable vs. Unstable Plaques

Not all plaques are equally dangerous. Some plaques are relatively stable, meaning they grow slowly and stay in place. Their fibrous caps are often thicker and not prone to rupture easily. These *Stable Plaques* may cause mild chest pain, but they do not always lead to heart attacks.

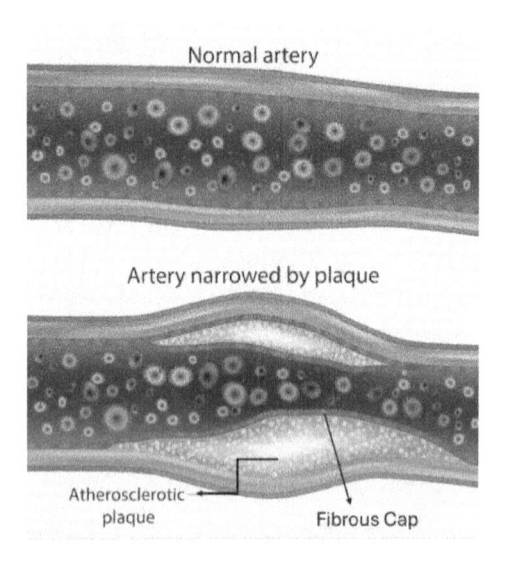

Fig. 10.1 Normal & Atherosclerotic Artery showing plaques

(Courtesy: Sakurra /Depositphotos.com)

However, other plaques are more dangerous because they are *unstable*. These *Unstable Plaques* (*vulnerable plaques*) can *rupture* (break open) unexpectedly. Often they have thinner fibrous caps which can tear easily. When a plaque ruptures, it triggers a chain reaction - the body's clotting system kicks in, forming a blood clot around the rupture site. If the blood clot is large enough, it can completely block the artery. When this happens, blood flow to that section of the heart is completely cut off and a heart attack occurs.

A heart attack, thus, is a medical emergency that begins with the blockage of a coronary artery, preventing oxygen from reaching the heart muscle supplied by that coronary artery. Recognizing the warning signs of a heart attack and seeking immediate treatment can help restore blood flow and prevent lasting damage to the heart.

Understanding the process (*Pathophysiology*) behind heart attacks highlights the importance of managing risk factors like high blood pressure, high cholesterol, and smoking, which contribute to plaque formation in the arteries and to the vulnerability and easy rupture of plaques.

Inflammation and Clot Formation

Let us see in a bit more detail what happens when a plaque ruptures.

A heart attack often starts with the rupture of a plaque. When the plaque breaks open, the fatty substances inside are exposed to the bloodstream. This sends a signal to the body that an injury has occurred—similar to how your body reacts when you cut your skin or suffer a burn.

Inflammation is the body's natural way of responding to injury. <u>Inflammation is a technical term which describes the body's immune system response to an irritant, such as a germ or foreign object, to fight infection or heal damaged tissue which has been injured</u>. When a plaque ruptures, the body sends *Platelets* to the area to help repair and seal the damage. However, in the arteries, this response can backfire. Instead of healing, the inflammatory response makes the area around the plaque rupture sticky, causing the tiny blood cells called *Platelets* to clump together at the site of rupture. This provides a nidus for a clot to develop and creates the ideal conditions for a blood clot to form.

The formation of a blood clot (*Thrombus*) is the crucial event that triggers a heart attack. As blood cells and proteins clump at the site of the ruptured plaque, a blood clot forms. This clot can grow large enough to completely block the artery, preventing oxygen-rich blood from reaching the heart muscle. The coronary artery in an adult has a diameter of only 3 -4 millimeters, and hence can get easily blocked by the clot.

To understand how this blockage affects the heart, think of it as a roadblock on a busy highway. When the road (the artery) is blocked, traffic (blood) cannot get through, and the areas beyond the blockage (the heart muscle) are deprived of essential items (oxygen). Without oxygen, the cells in that part of the heart begin to die.

Chronic inflammation can make plaque more likely to rupture in the first place. People with conditions such as diabetes, obesity, or those who smoke often have higher levels of inflammation in their bodies. This constant state of inflammation weakens plaques, making them unstable and prone to rupture. These are called the '*Vulnerable plaques*'. As a result, people with chronic inflammation are at a higher risk of having a heart attack.

Ischemia, Injury and Infarction

The heart, like any muscle, requires oxygen to function, and a blockage in the blood supply deprives heart muscle cells of this essential oxygen. When one of the heart's main coronary artery becomes blocked, the flow of blood to the area of the heart it supplies is reduced or cut off. This means that part of the heart muscle does not get enough oxygen and nutrients. This shortage of blood supply is called *Ischemia*.

When the blockage continues, the cells in the affected area suffer *Injury* initially and begin to lose function—they cannot contract properly. If the flow is not restored quickly, these cells die—a process known as *Infarction*. *Infarction*, meaning tissue death due to inadequate blood flow, is why a heart attack is medically referred to as a *Myocardial Infarction*, with "*myocardial*" referring to the 'heart muscle'. The area deprived of oxygen becomes the "*Infarct zone*," where heart muscle cells progressively die. If the blockage persists, the infarct zone expands, spreading the damage and increasing the risk of severe complications. Thus we see that when the blood supply is cut off, the affected part of the heart muscle progressively goes through the three phases: *ischemia*, *injury*, and then *infarction*.

The extent of the damage thus depends on how long the artery is blocked and how quickly treatment is received. If blood flow is restored soon after the heart attack begins, much of the heart muscle can be saved, the injury minimized, and the size of the infarct zone reduced. However, if the blockage persists for too long, the damage becomes permanent and extensive.

Unlike other tissues in the body, heart muscle tissue cannot regenerate after it is damaged. Once heart muscle cells die, they are replaced by *Scar Tissue* just as a scar forms when we are injured. Scar tissue cannot contract or pump blood as well as healthy heart muscle, which weakens the heart's ability to function properly. This means that any damage caused by a heart attack is permanent, and the heart will never fully regain its previous strength.

Consequently, the heart may not be able to pump blood as efficiently as it should. The heart becomes weak and its capacity to pump decreases. This condition is called *Heart Failure*, where the heart struggles to pump blood to meet the body's needs. Heart failure can lead to various symptoms like fatigue, shortness of breath, and a reduced ability to perform everyday activities.

In some cases, the damaged heart muscle can also interfere with the heart's electrical system, leading to abnormal heart rhythms known as *Arrhythmias*. These irregular heartbeats can be life-threatening if not treated promptly, as they can cause the heart to stop beating effectively.

Importance of Quick Action

Hence, the faster a heart attack is treated, the better the chances of saving heart muscle and preventing long-term damage. Recognizing the early signs of a heart attack—such as chest pain, shortness of breath, or discomfort in the arms, back, or jaw—and seeking immediate medical help can make a huge difference. Time is critical because the longer the heart goes without oxygen, the more damage is done.

Several treatments can help restore blood flow to the heart after a blockage. These will be discussed later. All these treatments work best when they are administered as soon as possible after the onset of a heart attack.

Silent Heart Attack

Not all heart attacks come with dramatic chest pain. Some people, particularly women or those with diabetes, can experience what is known as a "silent heart attack." Or *"Silent Myocardial Infarction"* (**SMI**). In these cases, the symptoms are mild or even absent, but the damage to the heart can still be significant. Silent heart attacks may go unnoticed at the time, but they still increase the risk of complications like heart failure or future heart attacks.

Thus a heart attack begins with the slow buildup of plaques in the arteries, a process that takes years to develop and eventually, these plaques can rupture, triggering the formation of a blood clot that blocks blood flow to the heart. Understanding how inflammation, clot formation, and oxygen deprivation contribute to a heart attack highlights the importance of managing risk factors like high blood pressure, high cholesterol, and chronic inflammation to protect your heart in the long run.

Key Takeaways

- *A heart attack (Myocardial Infarction) occurs when blood flow to the heart muscle is blocked, depriving it of oxygen, and causing potential damage or death to heart cells.*
- *The heart receives oxygen-rich blood through the coronary arteries; blockages in these arteries result in oxygen deprivation and damage to the heart muscle.*
- *Plaque buildup in the arteries, known as 'Atherosclerosis', is a gradual process that can lead to heart attacks when the plaque ruptures and triggers clot formation.*
- *Stable plaques cause less risk, while unstable plaques are prone to rupture, which leads to a blood clot that can fully block an artery.*

- *Inflammation, a response to plaque rupture, contributes to blood clot formation, increasing the risk of complete artery blockage.*
- *The extent of heart damage during a heart attack is directly related to how quickly the artery blockage is cleared; early treatment can minimize damage.*
- *Scar tissue replaces the damaged heart muscle, weakening the heart's ability to pump blood, which may result in heart failure or arrhythmias.*
- *Chronic inflammation, smoking, high blood pressure, and high cholesterol are risk factors that increase the likelihood of plaque rupture and heart attack.*
- *Silent heart attacks, often without obvious symptoms, can still cause significant heart damage and increase the risk of complications.*
- *Time is crucial in treating heart attacks—quicker intervention helps save heart muscle and reduce long-term complications.*

Chapter 11 SYMPTOMS OF HEART ATTACK

Recognizing the symptoms of a heart attack is crucial for saving lives, yet many people are unaware that heart attacks can present in various ways. While chest pain is the most well-known sign, heart attacks can also cause more subtle symptoms like shortness of breath, nausea, sweating, or even fatigue. These signs may vary between men and women, and some individuals, especially the elderly or those with diabetes, might experience atypical symptoms such as back or jaw pain.

This chapter will guide you through the common and less obvious symptoms of a heart attack, stressing the importance of quick recognition and response. Knowing these symptoms is vital to prompt immediate action. Understanding these warning signs could make all the difference in saving a life.

A heart attack can happen suddenly and without warning but recognizing the signs can save a life. Many people know that chest pain is a common symptom, but heart attacks can manifest in different ways, with some symptoms being more subtle or even atypical. Let us go over the most common and lesser-known symptoms of a heart attack, as well as explain why quick action is crucial to minimize damage to the heart.

Common Symptoms
Chest Pain or Discomfort

Chest pain or discomfort is the most well-known symptom of a heart attack. Most people describe it as a feeling of pressure, squeezing, fullness, or heaviness in the chest. This discomfort often occurs in the center or left side of the chest. Some individuals liken the sensation to *"an elephant sitting on my chest."* The pain may come and go, but during a heart attack, the discomfort typically lasts for more than a few minutes and unlike in angina, does not improve with rest.

The pain is not always limited to the chest. It can spread (*radiate*) to other parts of the upper body, including the arms (especially the left arm), shoulders, back, neck, jaw, or even the upper part of the abdomen. This happens because the nerves from the heart and other areas share the same pathways, causing pain to radiate to different parts of the body.

Shortness of Breath

Feeling out of breath, especially during rest or with mild activity, is another common symptom of a heart attack. This may begin suddenly and occasionally worsen over time. Sometimes, shortness of breath occurs with chest pain, but it can also happen without it.

When the heart is not getting enough oxygen due to a blocked artery, it struggles to pump blood efficiently to the rest of the body, including the lungs. This can make it difficult to breathe properly, even when one is not exerting oneself.

Nausea and Vomiting

Many people mistake a heart attack for indigestion because it can cause nausea, an upset stomach, or even vomiting.

The *Vagus nerve*, which connects the brain to the stomach, also plays a role in the functioning of the heart. During a heart attack, this nerve can be triggered, leading to symptoms like nausea or a burning sensation in the chest that resembles heartburn.

Sweating

Breaking out into a cold sweat is another classic symptom of a heart attack. Many people describe this as feeling clammy or sweaty, even in cool environments. Sometimes the sweating is so profuse as to drench one's clothes.

When the body is under stress, such as during a heart attack, it releases stress hormones like adrenaline through stimulation of the *Sympathetic Nervous System* (**SNS**). Stimulation of the SNS can release adrenaline and cause sweating. The body reacts by trying to cool down, which results in sudden, excessive sweating.

Dizziness or Lightheadedness

Some people may feel dizzy, lightheaded, or as though they might pass out. This can happen if the heart is not pumping enough blood to the brain, causing a drop in blood pressure thereby reducing the blood being pumped into the brain. This leads to a feeling of faintness.

This is a dangerous symptom. Dizziness or lightheadedness is a serious sign that blood flow to the brain has been disrupted. If untreated, it can lead to fainting or other life-threatening complications especially if the person is engaged in some crucial activity like driving or handling machinery.

Uncommon (Atypical) Symptoms

While the typical chest pain is the most common symptom of a heart attack, some people, particularly women, the elderly, or those with diabetes, may experience less obvious or *atypical* symptoms. Chest pain may not occur in them. These atypical symptoms can make it harder to recognize a heart attack, but they are just as important to know about.

Back Pain

Some individuals, especially women, may feel pain or discomfort in the upper back, often between the shoulder blades. This can feel like an ache, sharp stabbing pain, or pressure.

Unlike typical back pain from poor posture or injury, this pain often appears suddenly and may worsen when lying down or taking deep breaths. If one experiences unusual back pain, especially alongside other symptoms, it is important not to ignore it.

> Stella, a 55-year-old secretary, who used to smoke, began feeling nauseous and vomiting while at work after having a bagel and a banana for breakfast. Initially, she thought her symptoms were due to the food, but as the nausea persisted and she became extremely fatigued, she was unable to continue working. Concerned, a colleague rushed her to the emergency department.
>
> At the hospital, the resident diagnosed her with Atypical chest pain, although her symptoms did not seem typical of a heart attack. However, an ECG revealed an infarction in the inferior wall of her heart. A Coronary Angiogram showed a complete blockage of her right coronary artery. An emergency angioplasty was performed by the cardiologist, and a stent was placed to restore blood flow.
>
> Stella recovered without complications and was discharged on the fifth day. She was advised to adopt a healthier lifestyle, quit smoking, and reduce her weight. A regular cardiac rehabilitation program helped her gradually return to her normal routine within a month. Stella was prescribed medications and instructed to attend regular follow-up checkups with her cardiologist to ensure ongoing heart health.

Jaw Pain

Pain in the jaw, usually on the left side, can be a sign of a heart attack. This pain can also radiate down the neck and shoulders, making it easy to mistake it for a dental problem or muscle strain. The patient is likely to dismiss this as a toothache and not seek timely medical help.

Jaw pain is a type of *'referred pain'*, meaning that the heart sends pain signals to other areas of the body because of shared nerve pathways just as chest pain can spread to the arms or back during a heart attack.

Fatigue

The sudden onset of extreme fatigue or exhaustion, especially in women and older adults, can be a subtle but serious sign of a heart attack. This fatigue may appear suddenly and last for days or even weeks before the heart attack actually occurs.

When the heart is not working efficiently, it struggles to deliver enough oxygenated blood to the rest of the body. This can make even simple tasks like walking or standing feel exhausting. If a person feels unusually tired without a clear reason, it could be a warning sign of an impending heart attack.

Silent Heart Attack

Some people, especially those with diabetes or older adults, may experience what is known as a 'silent' heart attack' or *'Silent Myocardial Infarction'* (**SMI**). In these cases, the symptoms are mild or vague, such as slight discomfort, shortness of breath, or fatigue, rather than the classic chest pain. Often these mild symptoms may be passed off as 'gas trouble' or 'indigestion'. Occasionally, there may be no symptoms at all, and the heart attack is recognized only when an ECG is taken for some other purpose.

Silent heart attacks are dangerous because the symptoms of a silent heart attack, if at all they occur, are easy to overlook and many people do not seek immediate medical attention. This delay can result in greater damage to the heart, as the lack of oxygen continues to harm the heart muscle unnoticed.

Recognizing the symptoms of a heart attack can make all the difference in saving a life. One should remember that women, the diabetic and the elderly may experience less typical symptoms such as back pain, jaw pain, extreme fatigue, or even a silent heart attack without severe pain. *Time is key*—if anyone shows any of these symptoms, one should not hesitate to call emergency services immediately.

Gender Difference in Symptoms

For men, the most common symptom of a heart attack is intense chest pain or pressure. Men tend to recognize these classic heart attack symptoms more easily because they match the well-known signs. Chest pain, along with shortness of breath, is often a clear signal that something is wrong, prompting quicker medical attention.

However, symptoms in women may be atypical and subtle with more chances of being missed or misinterpreted. While chest pain is also common in women, it is often less intense or described as more of a pressure or tightness rather than sharp pain. Atypical symptoms, such as nausea, vomiting, pain in the back or jaw, and extreme fatigue may occur in women, and this can make it harder for women to recognize they are having a heart attack.

Also, women frequently report sudden and unexplained fatigue or shortness of breath, sometimes days before the heart attack. This may feel like an overwhelming tiredness, as if even small tasks are exhausting. Since these symptoms can be mistaken for stress or other everyday issues, many women may ignore them, not realizing they are signs of a heart attack.

Because women's symptoms are often more subtle or do not fit the classic description of a heart attack, they are more likely to be misdiagnosed or to delay seeking treatment. This delay increases the risk of severe heart damage or death, as early treatment is essential for minimizing the impact of a heart attack.

The differences in how men and women experience heart attack symptoms can lead to dangerous delays in treatment. Women, in particular, may wait too long to seek help because their symptoms do not seem serious or typical of a heart attack. This delay can result in more extensive damage to the heart.

Hence, it is crucial for both men and women to recognize that heart attack symptoms can vary. Knowing the less obvious signs—like jaw or back pain, fatigue, or nausea—can help ensure that medical help is sought immediately, which can prevent serious complications and save lives.

Importance of Quick Recognition and Response

When a heart attack occurs, every minute counts. The longer the heart is deprived of oxygen, the more muscle tissue is damaged. The damage can be permanent if treatment is delayed, making quick recognition and action vital to saving heart muscle and reducing long-term effects.

The first hour after a heart attack begins is often referred to as the *"Golden hour."* This is the critical window of time when immediate treatment like an angioplasty can greatly reduce heart muscle damage and improve the chances of survival. Quick medical intervention within this hour can minimize the extent of heart muscle injury and lead to a better recovery.

What to do if you suspect a Heart Attack

If you suspect that you or someone else is having a heart attack, the most important thing to do is call for emergency medical help right away. Do not wait to see if the symptoms go away spontaneously. It is always desirable to err on the side of safety. Time is of the essence, and every minute without treatment increases the risk of severe damage.

If you can, chew an aspirin while waiting for medical help to arrive. Aspirin helps to thin the blood, which can reduce the size of the clot blocking the artery. This can improve blood flow to the heart and lessen the severity of the heart attack. But one should be aware that some persons are allergic to aspirin and some people having stomach ulcer may not tolerate aspirin.

If you are having a chest pain, it is important not to drive yourself to the hospital, as you could lose consciousness while driving. Instead, call an ambulance. [See Chapter 13 on *Prehospital Management of Heart Attack*].

Recognizing the symptoms of a heart attack, especially the less typical ones, is important to ensure quick and effective treatment. While chest pain is the most common sign, other atypical symptoms may also indicate a heart attack, particularly in women. Understanding that symptoms can differ between men and women is essential, as is knowing what to do if you suspect a heart attack.

Key Takeaways

- *Chest pain or discomfort is a hallmark symptom of heart attack but can spread to other areas like the arms, shoulders, back, neck, or jaw.*
- *Shortness of breath, with or without chest pain, is a common warning sign caused by the heart's reduced ability to pump oxygenated blood.*
- *Other symptoms like nausea, vomiting, cold sweats, and dizziness can be mistaken for less severe issues but may signal a heart attack.*
- *Atypical symptoms, such as back or jaw pain and extreme fatigue, are more common in women, the elderly, and people with diabetes, often leading to delays in seeking help.*
- *Silent heart attacks, which can occur without noticeable symptoms, are especially dangerous and may only be detected through routine ECGs.*
- *Quick recognition of symptoms and immediate medical intervention are critical to minimizing heart damage, especially within the first "Golden hour."*

Chapter 12 DIAGNOSIS AND INVESTIGATIONS

Diagnosing a heart attack quickly and accurately is vital to saving lives and minimizing heart damage. This chapter explains the essential tests used by doctors to confirm a heart attack and assess its severity. An electrocardiogram (ECG) is often the first test, detecting abnormal heart rhythms and identifying affected areas of the heart. Blood tests, such as troponin level measurements, reveal heart muscle damage. Imaging tests, including echocardiograms and angiograms, provide detailed views of the heart and its blood vessels, helping doctors decide on the best course of treatment. The chapter helps patients understand what these test are, how these tests work and empowers them to make informed decisions and seek timely medical help.

Diagnosing a heart attack quickly and accurately is critical to saving lives. When a heart attack is suspected, doctors use a variety of tests to confirm the diagnosis and assess the extent of the damage to the heart. These tests help determine the best course of treatment, from medication to surgery, and can significantly impact the patient's recovery. Below we shall discuss the most common tests used to diagnose a heart attack and how they help doctors make decisions about care.

Tests Used in Diagnosis
Electrocardiogram (ECG)

An Electrocardiogram (**ECG**) is one of the first tests performed when a heart attack is suspected. It measures the electrical activity of the heart and helps doctors identify problems with the heart's rhythm and damage to heart muscle.

The heart's electrical system controls how it beats. During a heart attack, this system can be disrupted. The ECG picks up electrical signals from the heart using small sensors (*electrodes*) attached to the skin, usually on the chest, arms, and legs. These sensors record the heart's electrical activity as a graph, which allows doctors to look for abnormalities in the heart's rhythm. A normal person's heart gives a particular pattern of ECG recording which is considered normal. When a heart attack occurs, damaging the heart muscle, this pattern is altered, and the doctor is able to identify the heart attack by the changes in the patterns.

When a heart attack occurs, not all of the heart tissue supplied by the blocked coronary artery dies right away. Instead, different areas are affected in varying degrees: some are deprived of blood (*ischemia*), others undergo *injury*, and some muscle tissue is permanently damaged (*infarction*). These three zones—*ischemia, injury,* and *infarction*—can be detected through changes in an ECG. The ECG records the heart's electrical activity graphically, designated as P, QRS, and T waves. By examining changes in these waves, doctors can determine the extent, severity and location of the heart damage, helping them assess the severity of the heart attack. This allows for better treatment decisions. Thus the doctor is able to tell whether the attack has affected the front portion of the heart (*Anterior*), the back (*Posterior*), the side (*Lateral*) or the underside (*Inferior*) of the heart. Based on the location of the infarct, the physicians designate infarctions as *Anterior Wall Infarction, Posterior wall Infarction* etc. [**Fig 12.1**]

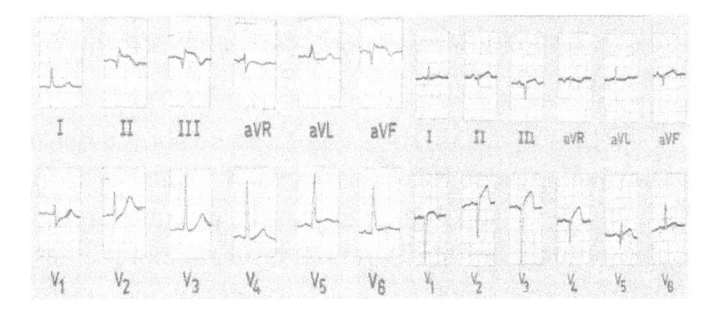

Fig 12.1. Two ECGs showing myocardial infarction.

The panel on the left shows infarction in the Inferior Wall (underside) of the heart. On the right shows infarction in the Anterior Wall (front) of the heart.

(**Images courtesy of the author from the book '*Understanding the Electrocardiogram*'**)

During a heart attack, the electrical signals that control the heartbeat can become irregular, which can be picked up in an ECG. This irregularity of the heart beat is called *Arrhythmia*.

Thus, the ECG is quick, painless, and provides results almost immediately, making it a crucial first step in diagnosing a heart attack. It gives valuable information to the treating doctors about the location and extent of the infarction.

Blood Tests (Troponin Levels)

When the heart muscle is damaged, as in a heart attack, certain proteins are released from the heart muscle cells into the bloodstream. The most important of these proteins is one called *Troponin*. Troponin is a protein found in heart muscle cells. When these cells are damaged, troponin leaks into the bloodstream. Normally, troponin levels in the blood are very low, but after a heart attack, they rise significantly.

Laboratory test of the patient's blood show a rise in troponin levels, and this is a strong indicator of heart muscle damage. The higher the levels, the more severe the heart attack. But the Troponin levels do not increase immediately after a heart attack starts. It can take several hours for troponin to show up in the blood, so doctors may repeat the test after a few hours to confirm the diagnosis. The amount of troponin in the blood helps doctors understand how much heart muscle has been affected and plan treatment accordingly. But the doctors may not wait for the tests to confirm infarction, if the ECG gives enough evidence regarding the heart attack, as time is of the essence in the treatment.

Imaging Tests

In some cases, doctors use imaging tests to get a clearer picture of the heart and its blood vessels. Two common imaging methods are *Echocardiogram* and *Angiography*.

Echocardiogram (Echo)

An *Echocardiogram* is an ultrasound examination of the heart. It uses high energy sound waves to create moving pictures of the heart in action. The echocardiogram shows the size and shape of the heart, as well as its chambers and valves. It reveals how well the heart is pumping blood, which is often affected during and after a heart attack. After a heart attack, the damaged parts of the heart muscle may not contract as the adjacent normal sections do. The doctor can see these areas on the screen of the monitor and can identify the areas of damage. It also helps in assessing the extent of damage to the heart muscle. [**Fig 12.2**]

An echocardiogram is usually performed after the initial tests, like the ECG and blood tests, to confirm the diagnosis and assess how much of the heart muscle has been damaged. It is a simple, painless, non-invasive test that provides important information about the heart's ability to function properly.

The amount of blood pumped out of the heart with each beat can be measured as a fraction of the total volume of blood in the left ventricle. This is called the *Ejection Fraction* (**EF**). The normal EF is 50–70%, meaning that 50–70% of the blood in the left ventricle is pumped out to the body with each heartbeat.

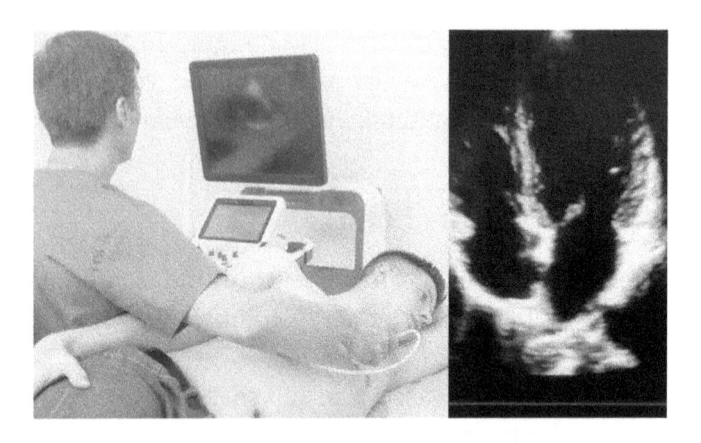

Fig 12.2 Echocardiography in Progress

The figure on the left shows the patient undergoing Echo. The figure on the right shows the four chambers of the heart

(Courtesy: Familylifestyle & Belish/Deposit photos)

When part of the heart muscle is damaged, the EF becomes low. A very low EF indicates that heart failure is developing.

The amount of blood pumped out of the heart in one minute is called the *Cardiac Output* (**CO**). This too can be measured using Echo. How the heart valves open and close and the various heart valve disorders can be made out. The size of the heart's chambers, including the left ventricle, right ventricle, and left atrium can be measured and the thickness of the heart's walls can be measured.

Angiography

Angiography is a procedure where the blood vessels are X-rayed after injecting a radio-opaque dye into them. The image thus obtained is called an *Angiogram*. When it is done to view the coronary arteries, it is known as a *Coronary Angiogram*. This test provides detailed images of the blood vessels in the heart.

During the procedure, a thin flexible tube called a *catheter* is inserted into an artery, usually in the arm or groin, and guided toward the heart into the coronary artery. A special dye is then injected into the bloodstream, making the coronary arteries visible on the X-ray. [**Fig 12.3, 12.4**]

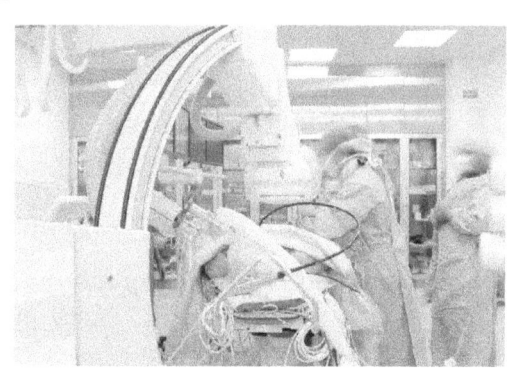

Fig 12.3. Showing Coronary Angiography in progress

(Courtesy: Sudok1 / Depositphotos)

The X-ray images reveal whether any of the coronary arteries are blocked or narrowed. The angiogram also shows how severe the blockages are, helping doctors decide whether treatments like angioplasty or surgery are needed. [See Chapter 15 on *Hospital Management of Heart Attack*].

Angiography is often performed during or after a heart attack to locate and treat the blocked artery. While it is an invasive procedure, it provides doctors with a clear view of what is happening inside the heart's blood vessels.

Once these tests are completed, doctors combine the results and analyze them to confirm whether a heart attack has occurred and to determine its severity. Here's how the different tests are used together.

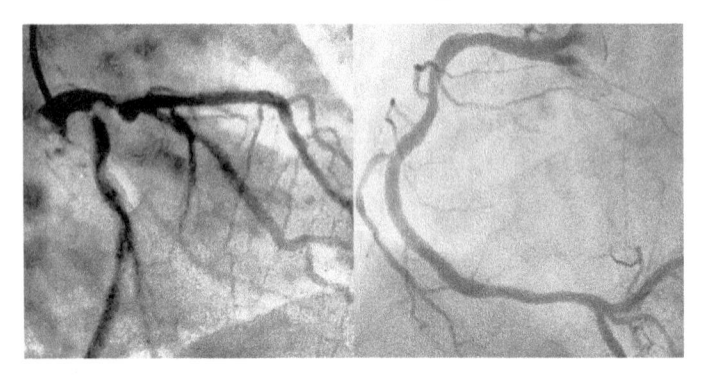

Fig 12.4. Coronary Angiogram

Figure showing Left Coronary Artery (Left) and Right Coronary Artery (Right) in the Coronary Angiogram image.

(Courtesy: Flik47 & Pitchayanank/ Deposit photos)

<u>Initial ECG</u>: The ECG is typically the first test performed. If it shows certain changes different from normal, doctors may immediately suspect a heart attack and perform further tests. Often the ECG confirms the diagnosis based on the pattern of changes. However, sometimes the ECG may appear normal or show only

minimal changes, especially in the early stages of a heart attack, even though the symptoms may be classical pointing to a heart attack. In such cases further testing is required and an ECG is repeated after some time.

Blood Tests (Troponin): Troponin levels play an important role in confirming the diagnosis. If the ECG does not suggest a definite heart attack and troponin levels are still low, doctors may monitor the patient and repeat the blood test and ECG after several hours. High troponin levels almost always indicate that heart muscle damage has occurred. This is done in doubtful cases.

However, if definite changes of a myocardial infarction are seen in an ECG, the doctors may proceed to performing an angiography and an angioplasty without much delay without waiting for troponin results. Often these tests are done simultaneously so as not to waste time, and a quick decision is taken regarding angiography which finally decides on whether angioplasty is needed or not.

Imaging Tests: If there is uncertainty from the ECG or blood tests, the echocardiogram can also provide a clearer picture of the heart's condition. It helps determine how much of the heart muscle has been affected by the heart attack. An Echo can be done at the patient's bedside and the results obtained immediately. Echo often shows that if there is reduction in blood flow to a part of the heart muscle, that section will not contract properly. This can be clearly made out in an echocardiogram.

In more severe cases, especially if immediate treatment is needed to open a blocked artery, angiography provides direct evidence of where the blockages are. This allows doctors to plan treatments like stenting or bypass surgery. Often, a combination of these tests are done immediately to arrive at a diagnosis.

These tests help doctors understand when the heart attack began, how much damage has been done, and which areas of the heart are affected. This information is crucial for them to determine the best treatment plan, whether it is medication to dissolve blood clots, angioplasty to open the arteries, or surgery.

Diagnosing a heart attack quickly is critical to saving lives and minimizing heart damage. By using a combination of ECG, blood tests, and imaging tests, doctors can confirm a heart attack and assess its severity. Each test plays an essential role in providing information about the heart's health and guiding the treatment approach. The sooner a heart attack is diagnosed and treated, the better the chances of recovery and preventing long-term damage to the heart.

Key Takeaways

- *An Electrocardiogram (ECG) is a crucial first step in diagnosing a heart attack, identifying abnormalities in the heart's electrical activity and revealing the location and severity of the attack.*
- *Blood tests, especially measuring troponin levels, are key in confirming heart muscle damage, as troponin levels rise significantly after a heart attack.*
- *Imaging tests like echocardiograms provide detailed pictures of the heart's function, showing*

areas of damage and assessing the heart's ability to pump blood.
- *Angiography helps visualize blockages in coronary arteries, guiding doctors in deciding if procedures like angioplasty or surgery are necessary.*
- *Combining results from ECG, blood tests, and imaging helps doctors confirm a heart attack, assess the damage, and choose the best treatment approach to minimize heart damage.*
- *Most of these tests are performed simultaneously so as not to waste time in managing the heart attack.*

Chapter 13 PREHOSPITAL CARE OF HEART ATTACK

A heart attack is a life-threatening emergency where quick and informed action can make all the difference in saving a life. In the critical moments before reaching the hospital, understanding the signs of a heart attack and knowing how to respond can reduce heart damage and increase survival chances. This chapter highlights the importance of calling emergency services immediately and taking steps to keep the patient calm while avoiding actions that could worsen the situation. Knowing when to offer aspirin, understanding what not to do, and ensuring professional medical help arrives swiftly can significantly improve outcomes during a heart attack.

A heart attack is a medical emergency and knowing <u>what to do and what not to do</u> before the person reaches the hospital can make a significant difference in saving their life. Every second counts when it comes to reducing damage to the heart and increasing the chances of survival. Let us go over the immediate actions to take when someone shows signs of a heart attack, why calling emergency services is critical, and what you should avoid doing to prevent worsening the situation.

Immediate Care
What to do if a person shows signs of a heart attack

When a heart attack strikes, the symptoms can be sudden and frightening. Recognizing these signs and acting quickly is key to saving a life. Here are the steps one should take to help the person with a suspected heart attack.

A heart attack usually comes with several warning signs, which are often the body's way of signaling that something is wrong with the heart. We have already discussed the symptoms of a heart attack in Chapter 11. Let us recapitulate them very briefly. Understanding these symptoms helps one act faster.

Chest pain: The most common symptom of a heart attack is chest pain or discomfort. This is often described as a heavy pressure, squeezing, or tightness in the center of the chest. The pain might feel as though there is a weight on the chest that will not go away.

Pain spreading to other areas: The chest pain can move to other parts of the body, including the arms (especially the left arm), neck, jaw, back, or stomach.

Shortness of breath: Difficulty breathing, even without chest pain, can occasionally be a sign of a heart attack. This happens because the heart is struggling to pump enough oxygen-rich blood to the rest of the body, leading to breathlessness.

Other symptoms: Some people may experience sweating, nausea, vomiting, dizziness, or sudden fatigue. They may feel clammy or lightheaded, and these symptoms should never be ignored, especially when paired with chest discomfort.

When a heart attack occurs, every minute is critical. The steps taken before the person reaches the hospital can make a significant difference in saving their life and reducing the severity of the heart damage. Let us see the basic first aid steps you can take, the role of *Emergency Medical Services* (**EMS**), and how they can improve the chances of survival during a heart attack.

Once you recognize that someone may be having a heart attack, as a bystander or onlooker, taking immediate action is critical. Some points in the Basic First Aid for the patient are noteworthy.

Keep the Person Calm - Offer Aspirin if Recommended

It is important for both the person experiencing the heart attack and anyone nearby trying to help him, to remain as calm as possible. Panic can increase heart rates and blood pressure, putting additional strain on the heart. Speaking calmly and reassuringly can help reduce anxiety for the patient. Stress and panic can make the situation worse during a heart attack. Keeping the person calm and as relaxed as possible can help reduce this strain, making it easier for the heart to function. This is of utmost importance.

Speak in a calm, soothing voice. Reassure them. Let the person know that help is on the way, and they are not alone. Reassuring them can lower their anxiety and help them feel more at ease.

Help the person into a comfortable position. Ideally, they should be sitting upright or in a reclined position, which reduces pressure on the heart and makes breathing easier. Avoid having them lie flat unless they feel faint. Advise them to take deep breaths, which helps to calm them.

Encourage the person to stay still and avoid sudden movements which could increase their heart rate. The goal is to keep the heart from working too hard while waiting for professional help.

Aspirin is commonly recommended in the early stages of a heart attack because it helps to thin the blood, which can reduce the severity of the heart attack by preventing further clotting. Offer aspirin only if the person is fully conscious and able to swallow without difficulty. If the person is drowsy or confused, it is safer to wait for the EMS. Make sure the person is not allergic to aspirin or has been told by their doctor to avoid aspirin as in patients with stomach ulcers. If you are not sure, it is better to wait for medical advice from professionals.

A heart attack occurs when a blood clot blocks an artery. Aspirin helps by thinning the blood, making it less likely to form more clots or enlarging the clot and allowing some blood to continue flowing through the narrowed artery.

The typical dose is one regular-strength aspirin (300-325 mg) or four low-dose aspirin (81 mg). Have the person *chew the aspirin* rather than swallowing it whole. Chewing helps the aspirin to be absorbed faster into the bloodstream, allowing it to take effect more quickly. The soluble form of aspirin named **Disprin 325** mg is available in India. This can be dissolved in an ounce of water and given to the patient to drink. It is rapidly absorbed and effective.

Avoid Certain Actions – the Don'ts

While waiting for help to arrive, there are certain things you should avoid doing, as they could make the situation worse.

- Don't allow the person to walk or move around. Any physical exertion can put added stress on the heart, which is already struggling to function properly. The best thing for the person to do is to sit or lie down in a comfortable position and remain as still as possible.

- Don't offer food or drinks. Even if the person says they are thirsty or hungry, avoid giving them anything to eat or drink. A few sips of water may be given. If their condition worsens and they become unconscious, there is a risk they could choke. So also, if they need an immediate treatment like an angioplasty, being on empty stomach is ideal. Some patients may vomit and there is a likelihood that the vomitus may enter the lungs.

- Don't drive them to the hospital. It may seem quicker to drive the person yourself, but it is far safer to wait for professional medical help. Paramedics can start treatment right away, which could be lifesaving, and they are trained to handle emergencies that may arise on the way to the hospital. In places or countries where immediate medical help may not be available, one should aim to get the patient to a good hospital as soon as possible.

- Don't wait to see if the symptoms will subside by themselves. It may lead to loss of precious time.

- Call for emergency medical help as soon as symptoms appear. Time is crucial in preventing permanent damage to the heart. Every minute counts and waiting to see if the symptoms pass could lead to further complications. So, *DON'T DELAY*.

Importance of Emergency Services

The first and most important step when someone shows signs of a heart attack is to call emergency services wherever they are available. The phone number to call them varies from country to country. Emergency medical personnel are trained to provide immediate care that can significantly improve the outcome for someone experiencing a heart attack.

Paramedics can begin life-saving treatment as soon as they arrive. They can provide oxygen to help with breathing, give medications to thin the blood or reduce pain, and, if needed, use a defibrillator to restore normal heart rhythm if the heart stops beating (*cardiac arrest*). These early interventions can prevent the heart attack from getting worse.

Getting to the hospital safely is another reason why calling an ambulance is important. Emergency personnel are equipped to handle sudden complications, such as *Cardiac Arrest* (when the heart stops beating), which can happen on the way to the hospital. Having medical professionals with the necessary equipment increases the chance of survival. But in places where ambulance services are not readily available, getting the patient to the hospital safely assumes priority.

Research has shown that people who call emergency services or reach a hospital at the earliest when having a heart attack have a better chance of survival compared to those who attempt to drive themselves or delay treatment. The sooner treatment begins, the more heart muscle can be saved, reducing the risk of long-term damage. Remember, "*Time is muscle*".

When you call emergency services, it is important to provide clear and accurate information so they can respond as quickly as possible.

Provide the exact address or location where you are. If you are in a large building or an unfamiliar area, give as many details as possible to help the paramedics find you quickly. Describe the symptoms the person is experiencing clearly, including how long they have been going on and whether they are getting worse. Mention if the person has chest pain, trouble breathing, or any other signs like sweating or dizziness.

If you know the person's medical history, share it with the emergency operator. This includes information like whether the person has had a heart attack before, if they have a known heart condition, high blood pressure, diabetes, if they have any allergies or if they are taking medications. This helps the paramedics prepare for what to expect when they arrive.

Knowing what to do in the critical moments before reaching the hospital can be the difference between life and death during a heart attack. Recognizing the symptoms early and calling emergency services immediately is the most important step in prehospital care. By acting quickly and calmly, you can help reduce the damage to the heart and increase the chances of a full recovery.

Emergency medical services (**EMS**) are essential in managing a heart attack before the patient reaches the hospital. They provide advanced care in the crucial minutes after a heart attack starts, increasing the chances of survival and reducing damage to the heart. Today most modern hospitals are equipped with emergency medical teams who respond to such calls immediately.

What EMS Teams Do

- ✓ When EMS team arrives, the first thing they do is assess the person's condition. They check vital signs, such as heart rate, blood pressure, and oxygen levels, to get an immediate understanding of how serious the situation is.
- ✓ They can get an ECG taken immediately and confirm the heart attack.
- ✓ If the person is having trouble breathing or their oxygen levels are low, paramedics may give them oxygen through a mask or tube. This helps ensure the heart and other organs get enough oxygen, which can prevent further damage.
- ✓ EMS teams are trained to give medications that can relieve pain and improve blood flow. For example, they may give *Nitroglycerin*, which helps to *dilate* (expand) the blood vessels, or additional aspirin if it has not already been taken. These medications can help stabilize the person until they reach the hospital.

- ✓ If the person's heart stops (*cardiac arrest*), EMS teams can use a *Defibrillator*, which delivers an electric shock to the heart to restore a normal heartbeat. Defibrillation is important because the sooner it is provided, the higher the chances of survival.
- ✓ While transporting the person to the hospital, EMS will continuously monitor their heart activity and vital signs. This allows them to respond immediately if the person's condition worsens on the way and ensures that the medical team at the hospital is ready to take over care the moment the patient arrives.
- ✓ EMS teams are equipped to provide treatment as soon as they arrive, which is much faster than if the person were driven to the hospital in a private car. This early treatment can be lifesaving and reduce the risk of long-term heart damage.
- ✓ EMS teams communicate with the hospital while en route, so the emergency room staff or heart specialists can be ready to act the moment the person arrives. This streamlines the process, ensuring that critical treatments, such as angioplasty, can begin as soon as possible. The cardiac catheterization laboratory can be kept ready by the time the patient reaches the hospital. The patient can be taken to the Cath. Lab without delay.

Thus the prehospital management of a heart attack is about acting quickly, staying calm, and knowing the right steps to take while waiting for professional medical help. Recognizing the symptoms of a heart attack, keeping the person calm, and offering aspirin (if appropriate) can help stabilize their condition. The role of emergency medical services (EMS) is vital, as they can provide life-saving treatments on the spot and ensure safe transport to the hospital. By following these guidelines, one can improve the patient's chances of survival and recovery during a heart attack.

Key Takeaways

- *Recognizing early symptoms such as chest pain, spreading pain, shortness of breath, and other warning signs is crucial for quick intervention during a heart attack.*
- *Staying calm and reassuring the person helps reduce stress, lowering their heart rate and blood pressure, which can prevent further strain on the heart.*
- *Position the person comfortably, preferably sitting upright, to ease pressure on the heart and facilitate breathing, while avoiding sudden movements to minimize heart strain.*
- *Administer aspirin if recommended, ensuring the person is conscious and able to swallow, as it helps thin the blood and reduce clot formation.*
- *Avoid physical exertion, food, and drinks, as these can increase heart strain or risk complications if the person loses consciousness or requires urgent procedures.*
- *Call emergency medical services (EMS) immediately for prompt care and transportation; paramedics can administer life-saving treatments like oxygen, medications, or defibrillation before reaching the hospital.*

- *EMS teams ensure continuous monitoring and prepare the hospital team for immediate action, improving survival chances and reducing heart damage.*

Chapter 14 EMERGENCY MANAGEMENT IN THE HOSPITAL

When a heart attack patient arrives at the hospital, rapid and effective treatment is critical to saving their life and minimizing long-term heart damage. This chapter focuses on the emergency procedures used to restore blood flow to the heart, such as clot-busting drugs, angioplasty, and stenting. The importance of quick intervention, particularly within the "Golden Hour," cannot be overstated—prompt action dramatically improves survival chances and reduces heart muscle loss. In addition to these life-saving treatments, medications to relieve pain, stabilize heart function, and prevent further clots are also vital.

When someone experiencing a heart attack arrives at the hospital, and the diagnosis has been confirmed, the medical team immediately begins treatment to restore blood flow to the heart and prevent permanent damage.

The priority goal is to quickly reopen blocked arteries and ensure the heart gets the oxygen it needs. We will discuss the emergency treatments doctors use to manage a heart attack, including clot-busting drugs, angioplasty, stenting, and medications that relieve pain and stabilize the heart.

Treatment in the Emergency Room

Once a person with a suspected heart attack reaches the emergency room, the focus is on prompt and effective treatment. Time is of the essence, as the longer the heart muscle is deprived of oxygen, the greater the damage.

Thrombolytics

Thrombolytics (Clot-Busting Drugs) are medications designed to dissolve blood clots that block the arteries in the heart. Blood clots are often the cause of heart attacks, as they obstruct the flow of blood, starving the heart of oxygen.

A heart attack usually occurs because a blood clot (*Thrombus*) forms inside one of the coronary arteries which cuts off blood flow, and without oxygen, the heart muscle begins to die. Thrombolytic drugs work by dissolving these clots, which helps restore blood flow to the heart muscle and reduces the amount of damage.

Thrombolytics are most effective when given as soon as possible after the onset of a heart attack, ideally within the first hour. The sooner they are administered, the better the outcome, as more heart muscle can be saved.

These drugs are often used when hospitals cannot immediately perform more advanced procedures, like angioplasty, and serve as a temporary but crucial treatment until more permanent solutions can be applied.

In many countries where immediate coronary angiogram and angioplasty cannot be performed owing to remoteness of the patient from a well-equipped hospital, thrombolysis or clot-dissolving technique is still used to tide over the crisis. Later when the patient is stabilized, he may be transferred to a higher center where advanced facilities are available.

While thrombolytics can be lifesaving, they come with a risk of causing excessive bleeding in other parts of the body. Though thrombolytics are easy to administer and easily available, there are many contraindications to their use like a recent surgery or stroke. Doctors carefully evaluate the patient to ensure they are safe candidates for this treatment. Some of the commonly available thrombolytics used are *Reteplase, Tenecteplase, Streptokinase* and *Urokinase*. These are administered intravenously either as an infusion or as a bolus injection.

Thrombolytics successfully dissolve blood clots in only about 50-60% of patients, which limits their effectiveness and makes them less ideal for treating acute myocardial infarction. However, they are valuable when immediate access to angioplasty is unavailable. While thrombolytics work to break down the blood clot itself, they does not address the plaque buildup inside the artery that partly blocks blood flow. This buildup, or plaque, can still cause new clots to form by rupturing. On the other hand, angioplasty provides a more complete solution by pushing this plaque against the artery walls, creating a clearer path for blood flow and opening up the blockage more effectively.

Angioplasty (Fig 14.1)

Angioplasty is a procedure used to physically open blocked arteries in the heart. It is a common and highly effective treatment for heart attacks, often performed as soon as possible to restore normal blood flow.

During angioplasty, the cardiologist inserts a thin tube, called a *catheter*, into a blood vessel, typically in the leg or arm. The catheter is guided into the coronary artery where there is a blockage.

Once the catheter reaches the blocked artery, a small, elongated balloon at the tip of the catheter is inflated under high pressure. This balloon expands and pushes aside the clot and any plaque buildup crushing it against the wall of the artery, allowing the blood to flow freely again.

Angioplasty is often the first choice for treating a heart attack when available because it provides a more direct and immediate way to restore blood flow than clot-busting drugs. It is most effective when performed within the first hour after symptoms start, known as the '*Golden Hour*'. Angioplasty has its known benefits.

- It significantly reduces the risk of long-term heart damage and improves the patient's chances of survival. Hence it helps limit the size of the infarction area.

- By reopening the artery and allowing blood to flow again, angioplasty can also help prevent future heart attacks by removing the blockage which the plaque had caused. Dissolving the clot using thrombolysis does not affect the plaque. It only dissolves the clot. But angioplasty addresses both the clot and the plaque.

- After an artery is reopened through angioplasty, doctors often place a *Stent* to keep the artery open. A stent is a small metal mesh tube similar to the spring in your ballpoint pen, that provides long-term support to the artery and ensures that blood continues to flow properly. The stent ensures that the arterial wall does not collapse once the balloon is removed. [**Fig 14.1**].

Once the balloon used in angioplasty is deflated and removed, the stent stays in place, acting as a scaffold to hold the artery open and prevent it from narrowing again. This narrowing again can rarely occur after angioplasty and is called *Restenosis*. Placing a stent at the site of opening the artery prevents this restenosis from happening.

There are various type of stents available. Some called *Bare-metal stents* are basic metal tubes that keep the artery open physically. Others are the *Drug-eluting stents* which are coated with a medication that is slowly released into the artery to prevent it from becoming blocked again by scar tissue or a new plaque.

ANGIOPLASTY

1. Stent with balloon inserted into blocked artery

2. Balloon inflated to expand stent

3. Balloon removed from expanded stent

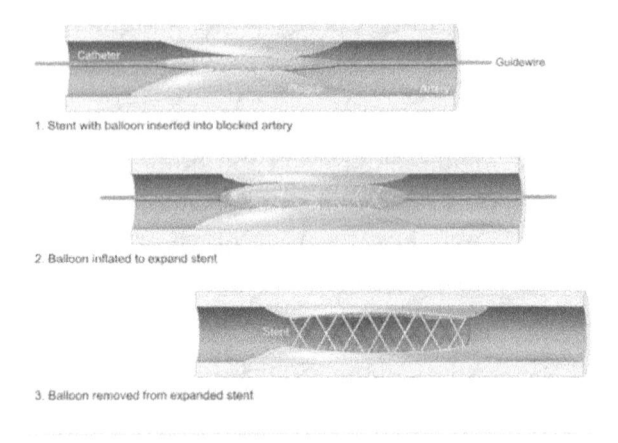

Fig. 14. 1. Angioplasty with Stenting

The figure shows 1. Stent with balloon inserted into blocked artery. 2. Balloon inflated to expand stent. 3. Balloon removed from expanded stent.

(Courtesy: Edesignua /Depositphotos.com)

Stents significantly reduce the chances of the artery becoming blocked again (*Restenosis*), lowering the risk of future heart attacks. Most patients who receive a stent will also need to take medications to prevent blood clots from forming inside the stent, ensuring that the artery remains open.

Emergency Medications

In addition to procedures like angioplasty and stenting, doctors use a variety of medications to help manage the symptoms of a heart attack and stabilize the patient's condition.

Medications to relieve the pain of a heart attack are administered to the patient. Some of these are:

Nitroglycerin: This medication helps widen (*dilate*) blood vessels, reducing chest pain and improving blood flow to the heart. It can also lower blood pressure, easing the strain on the heart. These can be administered as oral tablets, under the tongue (*sublingual*) or intravenously depending on the need.

Morphine: For severe chest pain, morphine may be used to reduce discomfort and help calm the patient. By reducing pain and anxiety, morphine can help lower the heart's workload.

Other medications: These are given to stabilize the heart. They are Beta blockers, Blood Thinners, Cholesterol lowering drugs and ACEI inhibitors, and are discussed in the next chapter on *Further Management in Hospital*.

Diuretics: If a patient is short of breath due to low levels of oxygen in blood or has fluid buildup in the lungs, they are given oxygen through a mask to help them breathe more easily. Additionally, medication to remove excess fluid from the body (*Diuretics*) is provided through an IV, working alongside the oxygen to relieve these symptoms.

In the emergency room, quick and effective treatment is essential for managing a heart attack. Procedures like angioplasty and stenting help restore blood flow to the heart, while medications like thrombolytics and beta-blockers reduce damage and stabilize the patient. The faster these treatments are administered, the greater the chances of saving heart muscle and improving recovery. By understanding the emergency management of a heart attack, we can appreciate the importance of immediate hospital care, and the life-saving procedures used to treat heart attack patients.

The Golden Hour
The Critical First Hour After a Heart Attack

When it comes to heart attacks, every second counts. The *Golden Hour* refers to the first 60 minutes after the onset of heart attack symptoms. This window of time is critical because the sooner treatment is given, the better the chances of survival and reducing permanent damage to the heart. That is why fast action within the golden hour can make the difference between life and death.

The heart muscle, which depends on oxygen to function, begins to die quickly without it. The longer the blockage remains, the more heart tissue is permanently damaged. This damage can weaken the heart, making it less effective at pumping blood throughout the body.

Hence, time is of the essence. If treatment is given during the golden hour, doctors can often restore blood flow to the heart and minimize the damage. But if this treatment is delayed, more heart muscle dies, leading to severe complications or even death. The quicker the blockage is treated, the better the chance of survival and recovery.

Consequences of Delayed Treatment

If treatment is delayed beyond the golden hour, the consequences can be life-altering. Acting within the golden hour also reduces the chances of developing serious complications. For example, when the heart muscle is severely damaged, it can lead to *Heart Failure* (when the heart becomes too weak to pump blood properly). This means that it becomes harder for the person to perform daily activities, exercise, or even walk short distances without becoming short of breath. Over time, this can severely affect the quality of life.

In some cases, delayed treatment can even cause sudden *Cardiac Arrest* (when the heart suddenly stops beating). Early treatment helps prevent these dangerous outcomes. Additionally, people who receive delayed treatment may be at higher risk for another heart attack or other heart-related complications in the future. This is why early recognition of heart attack symptoms and getting immediate medical help is so crucial.

Public Awareness of the Golden Hour

One of the biggest challenges in treating heart attacks is that many people do not recognize the symptoms quickly enough or delay seeking help. This is why public awareness is so important. Educating the public about the warning signs of a heart attack and the importance of acting quickly can save lives. The public should be educated that in a heart attack every minute counts. In short, the *Golden Hour* is not just a figure of speech—it is a race against time to save the heart. With faster treatment, we can give people the best possible chance for a full recovery and a healthy future.

Key Takeaways

- *Quick treatment in the emergency room is vital to restore blood flow to the heart and prevent long-term damage during a heart attack.*
- *Thrombolytics, or clot-busting drugs, are used to dissolve blood clots blocking arteries, but they are most effective when administered early, within the first hour.*
- *Angioplasty is a preferred procedure to physically open blocked arteries, often coupled with stenting to keep the artery open and prevent future blockages.*
- *Emergency medications like nitroglycerin, beta-blockers, and antiplatelets help reduce pain, improve blood flow, and stabilize heart function.*
- *The "Golden Hour" refers to the critical first 60 minutes after a heart attack when rapid treatment significantly improves survival rates and reduces heart muscle damage.*
- *Delayed treatment increases the risk of severe complications, including heart failure and future heart attacks, emphasizing the importance of immediate hospital care.*

Chapter 15 FURTHER MANAGEMENT IN HOSPITAL

After surviving a heart attack, hospital management focuses on stabilizing the patient and preventing further complications. This chapter outlines the critical steps taken in the hospital to monitor the heart's condition, manage potential risks like arrhythmias or blood clots, and begin the recovery process. Patients are closely observed in specialized units like the ICU, where continuous monitoring helps detect any issues early. Medications such as blood thinners, statins, and beta-blockers are prescribed to reduce the risk of another heart attack. This period is essential for empowering patients to take control of their health through proper care and prevention strategies for the future.

Once a heart attack has been treated, the road to recovery continues with careful hospital management.

The days following the heart attack are critical for monitoring the patient's condition and preventing further complications. Patients are often admitted to specialized units within the hospital where they are closely observed, and treatment is adjusted as necessary to promote healing and prevent future heart problems.

Monitoring in the Intensive Care Unit

After a heart attack, most patients are taken to the Intensive Care Unit (**ICU**) or a specialized heart care unit – the *Coronary Care Unit* (**CCU**). This is a controlled environment where doctors and nurses can keep a close watch on the patient's vital signs and recovery, especially in the critical hours and days after the event. The heart, having gone through severe stress, remains vulnerable, and close monitoring is essential to detect any complications early.

In the ICU, patients receive round-the-clock care from a dedicated team of healthcare professionals. This continuous monitoring is crucial because complications can arise quickly and need immediate attention.

Heart monitors: The patient's heart activity is constantly tracked using an electrocardiogram (**ECG**) which is displayed on a bedside electronic monitor. This device displays the heart's rhythm and helps detect any irregularities that could signal new problems, such as abnormal heartbeats or signs that the heart is struggling. [**Fig 15.1**].

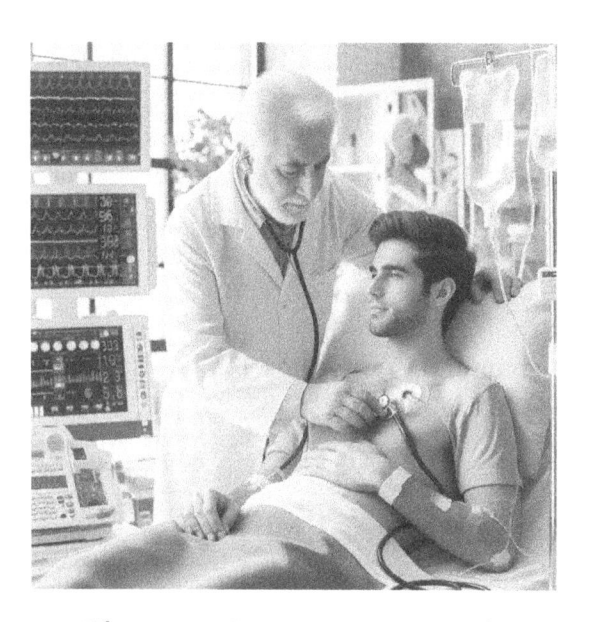

Fig 15.1. Coronary Care Unit

Patient in the Coronary Care Unit with various parameters being monitored using multiple equipment.

Blood pressure and oxygen levels: Vital signs like blood pressure and the amount of oxygen in the blood are also closely watched using appropriate equipment. Maintaining normal blood pressure ensures that the heart is not being overworked, while oxygen levels show if the heart is delivering enough oxygen throughout the body. The patient's breathing is also monitored, and the rate of breathing watched. Any sudden increase in the rate of breathing (*respiration*) indicates impending breathlessness and complications like acute heart failure.

Frequent blood tests: Regular blood tests are performed to measure specific substances, like *Troponin* (a protein released when the heart muscle is damaged), which helps doctors assess how much damage the heart has suffered and whether it is healing properly. The electrolytes in blood like sodium, potassium and magnesium are also monitored as changes in these electrolytes can lead to complications like arrhythmias or fall of blood pressure. For example, low sodium levels can lead to a drop in blood pressure, while abnormal potassium levels—whether too low or too high—can cause arrhythmias.

Potential complications

Some of the complications which are likely to occur while the patient is in the ICU during the early stages of a heart attack are enumerated below.

Arrhythmias: After a heart attack, patients can develop *arrhythmias*, which are abnormal heart rhythms. While some arrhythmias are harmless, others can be life-threatening, requiring immediate treatment. Medications or, in severe cases, electrical shock (*defibrillation*) may be used to restore normal heart rhythm.

Heart failure: If the heart has been weakened significantly by the heart attack, it may not be able to pump blood efficiently. This condition, known as *Heart Failure* (**HF**), can cause symptoms like shortness of breath and accumulation of fluid in the legs causing swelling. Acute heart failure is called *Acute Pulmonary Edema* when fluid suddenly accumulates in the lungs and the patient feels extremely breathless. ICU staff closely monitor for signs of heart failure to adjust treatments and avoid further damage.

Blood clots: There is an increased risk of developing blood clots after a heart attack. These clots can form in the left ventricle of the heart, the damaged arteries or in the veins and may lead to another heart attack or stroke if not treated promptly. Blood-thinning medications are often used in the ICU to reduce this risk. [See Chapter 16 on *Complications of Heart Attack*].

Medications to Prevent Future Heart Attacks

After the immediate danger has passed, the next step in hospital management is preventing future heart attacks. This is done through a combination of lifestyle changes and medications. Doctors will prescribe medications aimed at managing the factors that caused the heart attack, such as high cholesterol, blood clotting, and high blood pressure.

Blood Thinners

One of the main causes of heart attacks is the formation of blood clots that block the arteries supplying blood to the heart. Blood thinners are medications that reduce the ability of blood to form clots, lowering the risk of another heart attack. These are of various types.

Antiplatelet drugs: Medications like *Aspirin, Clopidogrel* or *Prasugrel* prevent platelets from sticking together and forming clots in the arteries. These are often prescribed after a heart attack to keep the blood flowing smoothly through the narrowed arteries.

Heparin: This is a type of blood thinner given to reduce the risk of new blood clots forming during and after treatments like angioplasty or thrombolysis. It is given as an injection.

<u>Anticoagulants</u>: Drugs like *Warfarin* or newer options such as *Dabigatran* work by interfering with proteins in the blood that are necessary for clotting. These drugs thus prevent blood from clotting. They are typically used for patients with a higher risk of blood clots inside the heart within the ventricle, but their dosage must be carefully managed to prevent excessive bleeding. They are also given to those patients in whom a clot has already formed inside the ventricle so as to prevent the clot from growing bigger.

Blood thinners and anticoagulants help keep the arteries open by preventing clots from forming. However, they must be used carefully because they can increase the risk of bleeding, so patients are closely monitored to ensure that the dosage is right for the patient.

Cholesterol-Lowering Drugs

High cholesterol is a major contributor to heart attacks. It leads to the buildup of fatty deposits (*plaque*) in the arteries, which can block blood flow. Statins are a class of medications that lower cholesterol levels in the blood and help prevent these blockages from forming.

Statins reduce the production of cholesterol in the liver, which in turn lowers the amount of cholesterol circulating in the bloodstream. By lowering cholesterol levels, statins help prevent plaque buildup in the arteries, reducing the risk of another heart attack.

Statins cannot remove existing plaques in the arteries, but they play an important role in making these plaques more stable, which helps prevent them from rupturing and causing a sudden heart attack. Additionally, statins can help stop the plaques from growing any larger.

The commonly prescribed statins are *Atorvastatin*, *Rosuvastatin* and *Simvastatin*. These medications are usually taken daily for the long term, perhaps for lifetime and studies have shown that they significantly reduce the risk of future heart attacks and strokes.

Beta-Blockers

Beta-blockers are medications that help reduce the workload of the heart by slowing down the heart rate and lowering the blood pressure. After a heart attack, the heart is often under extra strain, and beta-blockers help relieve this pressure.

By slowing down the heart rate, beta-blockers reduce the amount of oxygen the heart needs, giving the damaged heart muscle a better chance to recover. They reduce the work of the heart. They also lower blood pressure, reducing the risk of future complications such as another heart attack or heart failure.

ACE Inhibitors and ARBs

Another group of medications that play a key role in heart attack recovery is inhibitors *Angiotensin-Converting Enzyme inhibitors* (**ACEI**) and *Angiotensin II Receptor Blockers* (**ARBs**). These medications help relax blood vessels and reduce the workload on the heart. ACE inhibitors and ARBs block a chemical that causes blood vessels to tighten (*constrict*). By relaxing the blood vessels, these medications make it easier for the heart to pump blood. They also lower blood pressure and reduce the risk of heart failure, especially in patients whose heart has been weakened by the heart attack.

Thus, after surviving a heart attack, further hospital management focuses on two critical areas - closely monitoring the heart for potential complications and preventing future heart attacks through medications. Monitoring in the ICU ensures that any sudden problems, such as arrhythmias, heart failure, or blood clots, are recognized immediately and treated promptly. This comprehensive approach gives patients the best chance at a full recovery and helps prevent future heart attacks.

Further Hospital Management

After surviving a heart attack, the immediate threat may have passed, but the journey toward recovery is just beginning. Hospital management during this phase focuses on closely monitoring the patient, assessing the extent of heart damage, and preparing for long-term recovery. Let us briefly see how doctors assess the heart's condition and the extent of damage to the heart muscle after a heart attack and guide the patient toward a healthier future.

Once a patient is stable after a heart attack, the focus shifts to understanding how much damage the heart has suffered. This helps doctors plan for ongoing treatment and create a recovery strategy tailored to the patient's needs. Assessing heart damage typically involves several key tests and measurements. This needs certain tests which tell the doctor regarding the condition of the heart and the extent of the damage.

Echocardiogram

One of the primary tools doctors use to evaluate the heart after a heart attack is an *Echocardiogram*. This is a non-invasive test that uses high frequency sound waves (*ultrasound*) to create detailed images of the heart. This has already been discussed under diagnosis of heart attack.

The echocardiogram reveals the size and shape of the heart and how well the chambers and valves are functioning. Most importantly, it shows which parts of the heart muscle may have been damaged by the heart attack. If a section of the heart is not contracting properly, it can be seen in the echocardiogram and indicate that this area has been weakened or damaged. An echocardiogram helps doctors get a clear picture of how much of the heart muscle has been affected, which is critical for determining the next steps in treatment.

Another key measurement doctors focus on is the *Ejection Fraction* (**EF**). This refers to the percentage (*fraction*) of blood in the left ventricle that the heart pumps out with each beat. The ejection fraction is an important indicator of how well the heart is working overall. This is calculated during the echocardiographic study. A healthy heart typically pumps out 50-70% of the blood in its chambers with each beat. This is considered a normal EF.

After a heart attack, the ejection fraction may decrease, showing that the heart is not pumping as efficiently as it should. A significantly reduced ejection fraction can be a sign of heart failure, a condition where the heart struggles to circulate enough blood to meet the body's needs. For example if the EF is 40%, the doctor understands that the patient's cardiac function is significantly impaired, and he is liable to develop the symptoms of heart failure. This helps the doctor take preemptive action to prevent the complications of a low EF.

Doctors also use advanced imaging tests like *Magnetic Resonance Imaging* (**MRI**), or CT scans to measure ejection fraction and assess how much the heart's ability to pump blood has been affected. But the Echo provides the easiest and cheapest way to measure the EF.

Stress Tests

To understand how well the heart functions during activity, doctors may recommend a *Stress Test*. This test evaluates how the heart performs under physical stress, which is helpful in determining how much of the heart muscle remains healthy and how much has been damaged. It also gives the patient an idea of the amount of physical activity he can undertake after discharge.

During a stress test, the patient is asked to walk on a treadmill or pedal a stationary bike while their heart rate, blood pressure, and ECG are carefully monitored. The doctors observe whether the ECG changes appear when the patient is subject to such physical stress. For patients who cannot exercise, doctors may use a medication that simulates the effects of exercise on the heart, causing it to work harder and faster as if under physical stress. The stress test helps doctors see how well the heart handles increased activity. It shows whether enough blood is flowing to the heart muscle, or if the patient experiences discomfort or signs of strain. If blood flow is limited, it may indicate more severe damage or the need for further treatment.

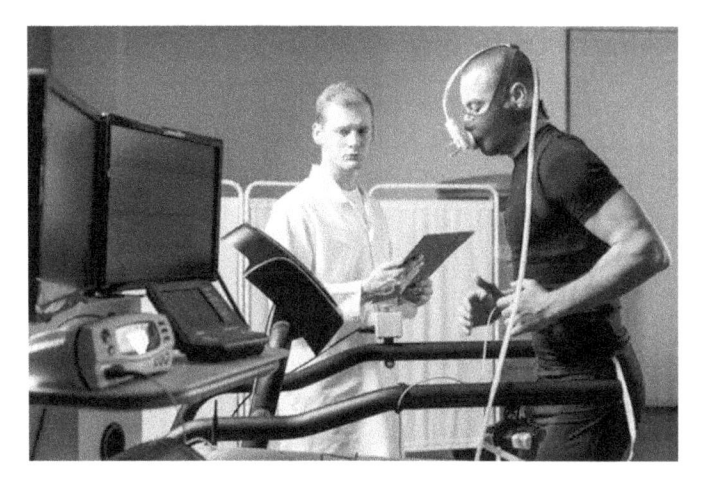

Fig 15.2. Treadmill Stress Test

Figure showing a patient walking on a Treadmill being monitored by the healthcare provider.

(Courtesy: Photographee/ Deposit photos)

Sometimes the stress test is performed before the patient is discharged from the hospital or later when the patient is asked to come after a couple of weeks. It is also performed as a part of the *Cardiac Rehabilitation* program. [see Chapter 18].

Preparing the Patient for Discharge

Once the patient's condition has stabilized, and doctors have assessed the heart damage, the focus shifts to preparing the patient for discharge from the hospital. This stage is crucial because it sets the foundation for a smooth recovery at home and helps prevent future heart attacks.

Developing a Recovery Plan

Before leaving the hospital, patients will be given a detailed recovery plan. This plan outlines medications, lifestyle changes, and follow-up care to ensure a successful recovery.

Medications: The patient's medications are thoroughly reviewed, and clear instructions are given on how and when to take them. Blood thinners, cholesterol-lowering drugs (like statins), ACE inhibitors and other heart medications will be a key part of long-term treatment.

Cardiac rehabilitation: Most heart attack patients will be enrolled in a *Cardiac Rehabilitation* program. Cardiac rehabilitation is a structured program that includes supervised exercise, educational sessions on heart health, and emotional support to help patients recover and regain their strength. This program is vital for improving heart health and reducing the risk of future problems. [See Chapter 17 on *Convalescence after a Heart Attack*].

Lifestyle Changes

Lifestyle changes are one of the most important aspects of preventing future heart attacks. These changes are aimed at improving overall heart health and managing risk factors like high blood pressure, cholesterol, and weight.

Diet: Doctors recommend adopting a heart-healthy diet that limits unhealthy fats, processed foods, and excessive salt. Instead, patients are encouraged to eat more fruits, vegetables, whole grains, and lean proteins. This helps lower cholesterol and blood pressure, which are key to preventing future heart attacks.

Exercise: Gradual and supervised physical activity is often advised. Patients may start with light exercises, like walking, and gradually increase the intensity as they recover and gain more strength. Regular exercise improves heart function and overall fitness.

Quitting smoking: Smoking significantly increases the risk of heart attacks. Patients who smoke are strongly encouraged to quit, and they will receive support such as counseling, medications, or nicotine replacement therapy to help them stop smoking. This change can greatly reduce the risk of future heart issues. [See Chapter 19 on *Lifestyle Changes after Heart Attack* and Chapter 20 on *Prevention of Heart Attack*].

Follow-Up Care

After discharge, follow-up care is essential to monitor the patient's progress and make any necessary adjustments to treatment.

Doctor visits: Regular appointments with the cardiologist will allow doctors to check how well the heart is healing and whether the medications are working effectively. These visits are crucial for tracking recovery and catching any potential problems early.

Monitoring symptoms: Patients are advised to be vigilant about any recurring symptoms, like chest pain or shortness of breath. If these occur, they should seek medical attention immediately to avoid further complications.

Further tests: The cardiologist may ask for further tests like an Echocardiogram to be repeated if the previous result had shown a low EF. This helps to assess if the patient's cardiac function is improving. Repeat ECG may be done to assess whether the previous ECG changes have regressed, or new changes have appeared. A stress test during the convalescence period may be done to assess whether the patient is capable of returning to his job. Blood tests are done regularly to monitor the cholesterol and blood sugar levels in those patients where they were high.

Summing up, recovering from a heart attack involves more than just surviving the initial event—it requires ongoing care and careful management to ensure a full recovery. As patients prepare to leave the hospital, they are given a detailed recovery plan that includes medications, lifestyle changes, and follow-up care. By following this plan and making healthy choices, patients can improve their heart health, reduce the risk of future heart attacks, and regain control of their lives.

Key Takeaways

- *After a heart attack, patients are closely monitored in the ICU to detect complications like arrhythmias, heart failure, and blood clots, ensuring prompt treatment.*
- *Continuous monitoring of heart function, blood pressure, and oxygen levels is essential for early*

detection of any issues, while frequent blood tests assess heart muscle damage.
- *Medications such as blood thinners, statins, beta-blockers, and ACE inhibitors are prescribed to prevent future heart attacks by managing blood clot formation, cholesterol, and blood pressure.*
- *Tests like echocardiograms and stress tests help evaluate heart damage and function, guiding long-term treatment plans for recovery.*
- *Patients are provided with a detailed recovery plan that includes lifestyle changes, medication adherence, cardiac rehabilitation, and follow-up care to ensure ongoing heart health and prevent future attacks.*
- *Lifestyle modifications like adopting a heart-healthy diet, regular exercise, and quitting smoking play a crucial role in long-term recovery and reducing the risk of another heart attack.*

Chapter 16   COMPLICATIONS OF HEART ATTACK

A heart attack can cause significant damage to the heart and other parts of the body, leading to a range of complications that affect long-term health. This chapter explores some of the most common complications that may arise after a heart attack, such as acute pulmonary edema, heart failure, and arrhythmias. Structural damage to the heart, like ventricular aneurysm, or critical conditions like cardiogenic shock can also occur. Additionally, heart attacks increase the risk of forming blood clots that can lead to strokes or blockages in other arteries. This chapter also emphasizes how these complications are treated, from medications and lifestyle changes to surgical interventions, empowering patients with knowledge to take an active role in their recovery and ongoing care.

A heart attack is a serious medical event that can leave lasting effects not only on the heart but also on the rest of the body. While modern treatments can save lives and reduce immediate damage, many people experience complications afterward. Understanding these complications is crucial for managing health and improving recovery.

After a heart attack, the heart may not function as well as it once did, and complications can arise that affect recovery and long-term health. Some of the complications like Acute pulmonary Edema and Arrhythmias may occur immediately while the patient is in the hospital whereas others like chronic heart failure or ventricular aneurysm may develop later. Here are some of the most common complications that can occur.

Acute Pulmonary Edema

Heart failure after a heart attack occurs when the heart cannot pump enough blood to meet the body's needs. It can be sudden in onset when it is called *Acute Pulmonary Edema* (**APE**) or *Acute Left Ventricular Failure*, or it can develop gradually and last for a long time when it is called *Chronic Heart Failure*.

Acute pulmonary edema is a life-threatening condition that occurs when the heart suddenly fails to pump blood effectively. This can happen as a result of a heart attack, where part of the heart muscle, specifically the left ventricle, is damaged. The left ventricle is the main chamber responsible for pumping oxygen-rich blood to the body. When it becomes weak, blood cannot be pushed forward into the aorta as it should. Instead, the blood backs up into the left atrium and then into the pulmonary veins, which are the blood vessels that bring oxygenated blood from the lungs to the heart.

As the pressure in these veins builds up, fluid from the blood leaks into the tiny air sacs in the lungs (*Alveoli*), leading to *pulmonary edema*. This accumulation of fluid in the lungs makes it very difficult for the patient to breathe, often causing sudden shortness of breath. Acute pulmonary edema is a medical emergency that requires immediate attention, as it can quickly lead to death if not treated.

In some cases, APE can occur not only because of a heart attack but also due to mechanical complications in the heart, such as a *Ruptured Papillary Muscle* (tiny muscles inside the left ventricle which help control the heart's valves) or a tear in the wall (*Septum*) between the heart's chambers. These problems further increase the amount of blood in the left ventricle, worsening the condition and leading to more fluid leakage into the lungs.

Symptoms of Acute Pulmonary Edema

The common symptoms of acute pulmonary edema include:

- Sudden shortness of breath, especially worse when lying down or during physical activity.
- A feeling of suffocation or drowning, particularly when lying flat. The patient tends to sit upright.
- Rapid, shallow breathing and gasping for air.
- Dizziness, fatigue, and excessive sweating.
- Coughing that may worsen as fluid builds up in the lungs. The patient may bring up pink, blood stained, frothy sputum.
- Anxiety and restlessness.
- In severe cases, the lips and skin may turn blue (*Cyanosis*) due to a lack of oxygen in the blood.

Diagnosis of Acute Pulmonary Edema

Doctors can often diagnose APE by listening to the patient's chest with a stethoscope. A characteristic crackling or bubbling sound, called *"rales,"* is heard, indicating fluid in the lungs. Additionally, the patient may appear sweaty, extremely short of breath, and have bluish lips, all signs that their body is not getting enough oxygen. The patient may cough up a pink, frothy sputum which is due to blood staining of the sputum.

A chest X-ray is commonly used to confirm the diagnosis, as it shows the fluid buildup in the lungs and other signs of pulmonary edema.

Treatment of Acute Pulmonary Edema

Immediate treatment is critical for APE. The primary focus is on treating the underlying cause, such as a blocked coronary artery during a heart attack. The goal is to restore proper blood flow to the heart as quickly as possible.

For immediate treatment of APE, oxygen therapy is provided to help increase the oxygen levels in the blood, typically delivered through a mask or nasal prongs. Medications called

> Fifty-five-year-old Edward, a chef at a five-star hotel, led a carefree lifestyle, enjoying good food, smoking around 10 cigarettes a day, and binge drinking on weekends. One Monday morning, while preparing breakfast for a valued customer, he suddenly experienced chest discomfort and shortness of breath. Within minutes, he started coughing up pink, frothy sputum, and his lips turned blue. Edward was rushed to the hospital, where he was diagnosed with Acute Pulmonary Edema. An ECG revealed a massive myocardial infarction in his left ventricle.
>
> He was immediately treated with intravenous medications and oxygen inhalation. An angiogram followed by an angioplasty was performed, saving his life. After a week in the hospital, Edward was discharged with medications and strict lifestyle recommendations. Determined to recover, he adhered to his new diet, quit smoking, and cut down on alcohol. Six weeks later, Edward returned to his kitchen, committed to living a healthier life.

Diuretics are administered intravenously to help the body get rid of the excess fluid in the lungs. These drugs work by making the kidneys produce more urine, which helps reduce the fluid buildup.

Other medications may also be used to strengthen the heart's pumping action and improve blood circulation. In severe cases where breathing becomes too difficult, the patient may need to be put on a *ventilator*. A tube made of polyvinyl chloride (PVC), or silicone is inserted into the windpipe (*Trachea*), and a machine helps pump a mixture of air and oxygen into the lungs.

With prompt treatment, many patients can recover from acute pulmonary edema, but it remains a serious condition that requires ongoing monitoring and care.

Chronic Heart Failure

Chronic Heart failure also called *Congestive Heart Failure* (**CHF**) is a condition that can develop when the heart muscle is too weak to pump blood effectively throughout the body. It often happens after a heart attack if a large portion of the heart muscle is damaged.

A heart attack damages part of the heart muscle, which reduces the heart's ability to pump blood. If enough of the muscle is affected, the heart cannot keep up with the body's demands for blood and oxygen. This leads to heart failure.

Symptoms of heart failure

<u>Shortness of breath</u>:   Patients may feel breathless during physical activity or even when resting or lying down, as the heart struggles to circulate oxygen-rich blood.

<u>Fatigue</u>:   A constant feeling of tiredness, even after mild activities, is common because the body is not getting enough oxygen. In severe heart failure, the exhaustion may be severe, and the patient is unable to carry out even his normal routine daily activities like looking after himself. Bathing, using the toilet and changing clothes may leave him exhausted.

<u>Swelling</u>:   Fluid can build up in the legs, ankles, or abdomen. This condition is called *Edema* and is caused by the heart's weakened pumping action which allows

fluid to accumulate in the tissues. The abdomen may become bloated, and the legs become heavy due to the accumulation of fluid.

In addition, others features like severe fatigue, decrease in urine output, low blood pressure, and confusion may be noticed.

Echocardiography, Chest X ray and some blood tests are used to confirm the presence of heart failure and assess the prognosis of the patient.

Management of Heart Failure

The following is a brief summary of how heart failure is managed.

General Measures: The patient is given light, nutritious diet. In the initial stages liquid diet may be needed. Salt is restricted to reduce the amount of fluid in the tissues of the body. The patient is kept as comfortable as possible. Many prefer to lie propped up in bed or a couch. While sitting, the feet may be elevated on a stool with a soft cushion under the heels. The temperature in the room should neither be too hot nor too cold. In hot climates when the ambient temperature is high, heart failure tends to be aggravated. Patients who have chronic heart failure are advised *Influenza* and *Pneumonia* vaccination.

Medications: *Diuretics* (water pills) are medications which help the body eliminate the excess fluid, reduce the swelling and ease the workload on the heart. *Beta-blockers* and *ACE inhibitors* are medications which lower blood pressure and help the heart pump more efficiently and thereby reduce the stress on the heart muscle.

Lifestyle changes: Adopting a heart-healthy diet, getting regular exercise, and quitting smoking are essential for managing heart failure.

Device Therapy & Surgery: Some patients may need devices like a pacemaker to help the right and left sides of the heart beat in synchrony. Others might require surgery, such as a *Coronary Artery Bypass* (**CABG**), to manage heart failure. Others may need replacement of a heart valve. In some cases, a mechanical support device called a *Ventricular Assist Device* (**VAD**) is used to pump blood from the weakened lower chambers of the heart to the rest of the body. For those with severe end-stage heart failure, a heart transplant from a brain-dead donor can provide significant benefits.

Monitoring and follow-up: Regular doctor visits help monitor heart function and adjust treatments as needed. In some severe cases, devices like pacemakers or surgery may be required to help the heart work better.

Mechanical Complications

Mechanical complications from a heart attack including the tearing (*rupture*) of the heart's wall, muscle, or internal structures, such as the valves can occur at times. These issues, though rare, can lead to severe consequences like internal bleeding or severe heart failure. Some examples include a rupture of the heart muscle, or the formation of abnormal bulging in the wall of the left ventricular wall called *Aneurysms*. Ventricular aneurysm will be dealt with in more detail. These conditions are life-threatening and require immediate medical attention, as they can quickly lead to death if not treated promptly.

Deformity and Compression of Cardiac Chambers

A heart attack can cause damage to the heart's walls, weakening the structure and leading to deformities

> Sarah, a 65-year-old woman living alone, was found slumped over her breakfast table one morning by her caretaker, who visited daily. Alarmed, the caretaker immediately called an ambulance. Sarah was rushed to the hospital, where doctors diagnosed her with a heart attack. She was admitted to the cardiac ICU, and an angioplasty was performed. On the third day of her recovery, Sarah suddenly collapsed, and her blood pressure dropped to dangerously low levels. A bedside echocardiogram revealed a life-threatening complication—her left ventricle had ruptured, causing blood to accumulate in the pericardium, compressing her heart. It was a Cardiac Tamponade.
>
> Immediately, Sarah was taken for emergency cardiac surgery. The surgeon discovered a half an inch tear in her left ventricle, which was carefully sutured. Thankfully, Sarah recovered well from the surgery. Although her hospital stay was prolonged, she experienced no further complications and was eventually discharged in stable condition.

or compression of the heart chambers. This makes it difficult for the heart to expand and pump blood properly. These changes can worsen heart failure, leading to symptoms like shortness of breath, fatigue, and swelling in the legs. Over time, this damage can significantly reduce the heart's overall function, requiring medical or surgical interventions to improve quality of life.

Ventricular Aneurysm

A ventricular aneurysm is a rare but serious complication that can occur after a heart attack. It happens when part of the heart's wall, particularly the left ventricle, becomes weak. The left ventricle is the main pumping chamber of the heart, and during a heart attack, damage to this part of the heart muscle can lead to the development of an aneurysm. This weakened area of the heart wall can bulge outward, much like a weak spot on a balloon expands and bulges out when filled with air. Every time the heart pumps blood, the aneurysm bulges outwards, increasing the risk of dangerous complications, such as rupture.

Ventricular aneurysms tend to develop after a severe heart attack, especially when the heart attack affects the full thickness of the heart muscle. The aneurysm does not form immediately but gradually appears as the heart tissue heals and forms scar tissue. Around 5% to 7% of people who have a heart attack go on to develop a ventricular aneurysm. Although it is a relatively rare condition, it is potentially life-threatening and requires careful monitoring.

Causes

As the heart heals, the dead muscle tissue is replaced by scar tissue, which is not as strong or flexible as the original muscle. Over time, this scar tissue can stretch and weaken, bulging outwards leading to the formation of an aneurysm. This weakened part of the heart wall becomes more vulnerable to complications.

Symptoms

The symptoms of a ventricular aneurysm may vary, but many patients experience breathlessness, especially during physical activity. Some may also feel palpitations, or the sensation of their heart racing or beating irregularly. This is because a ventricular aneurysm can lead to abnormal heart rhythms, known as *arrhythmias*, which can sometimes be dangerous. In severe cases, patients may develop heart failure, a condition where the heart is no longer able to pump blood efficiently, leading to fatigue, swelling, and difficulty breathing. Deaths from ventricular aneurysms are often caused by heart failure, arrhythmias, or the formation of blood clots in its walls (*Mural Thrombus*). These clots may dislodge and be carried into different parts of the body to block the blood vessels in different vital organs of the body. These clots arising from the heart and traveling to other parts of the body are called *Emboli*. (Sing: *Embolus*).

Ventricular aneurysms can be diagnosed using Echocardiography, Chest X ray or Cardiac MRI.

Treatment

Treatment for ventricular aneurysm depends on how severe the condition is and whether it is causing significant symptoms. For some patients, medications can help manage symptoms and reduce the risk of complications. These medications may include drugs to regulate the heart rhythm (*Anti-arrhythmic drugs*), reduce the workload on the heart, or prevent blood clots from forming (*Anticoagulants*).

In more severe cases, especially when the aneurysm poses a high risk of rupture or is causing significant symptoms like heart failure, surgery may be necessary. Surgical options may include removing the aneurysm surgically and repairing the damaged area of the heart.

With proper management and treatment, many patients with ventricular aneurysms can live longer and healthier lives, but ongoing medical supervision is essential.

Arrhythmias

Arrhythmias are irregular heartbeats that can develop after a heart attack because of damage to the heart's electrical system. These irregular rhythms can range from mild to life-threatening. They may cause the heart to beat too rapidly (*Tachycardia*), too slowly (*Bradycardia*), or erratically. The heart's electrical system controls the normal rhythm of the heartbeat which is regular at approximately 70 beats a minute. When a heart attack damages this system, it can cause the heart to beat irregularly.

Arrhythmias can lead to symptoms like dizziness, shortness of breath, fainting, or sudden cardiac arrest, where the heart stops pumping blood effectively. Proper medical treatment is essential to manage these conditions.

Types of arrhythmias

Various types of arrhythmias occur as a complication of heart attack. We shall discuss a few of them in brief.

Atrial fibrillation (**AFib**): A common arrhythmia where the upper chambers of the heart (*Atria*) beat *irregularly* and too fast, increasing the risk of stroke and heart failure. The heart rate may rise to very high levels of 150 or 160 per minute.

Ventricular tachycardia (**VT**): This is a fast but *regular* abnormal heartbeat that occurs starting in the lower chambers of the heart (*Ventricles*). If not treated, VT can lead to more serious issues like ventricular fibrillation.

Ventricular fibrillation (**VFib**): This is the most dangerous arrhythmia, where the heart quivers instead of pumping blood effectively. There are no effective beats and the ECG or monitor shows only an irregular wavy line. VFib requires immediate treatment, as it causes sudden cardiac arrest and if untreated, the patient dies.

Heart Block: Certain arrhythmias can cause the heart to beat too slowly or irregularly. One common type is called a *"Heart Block,"* which happens when the heart's natural electrical signals arising from the *Sinus Node* are delayed or blocked as they move from the upper (*Atria*) to the lower chambers (*Ventricles*). This disruption slows down the heartbeat because the signals do not reach the entire heart in a steady way. Heart blocks are often classified by how severe the delay is. In a mild case, signals might simply be delayed (*First-degree block*), but in more serious cases (*Second- or Third-degree blocks*), some signals may not get through at all, causing the heart to beat very slowly.

Complete heart block (**CHB**) or *Third-degree heart block* is a condition where the heart's electrical signals cannot travel from the upper chambers to the lower chambers, causing them to beat independently. The upper chambers continue at about 70 beats per minute, while the lower chambers slow down to 20-40 beats per minute. This can lead to tiredness, dizziness, or even fainting, since the body is not getting enough blood flow with each beat.

Cardiac Arrest: Cardiac arrest is a serious health emergency that occurs when the heart suddenly stops beating, preventing blood from flowing to the brain and other organs. Cardiac arrest is dealt with in detail below.

Symptoms of arrhythmias:

Palpitations: The sensation that the heart is racing, pounding, or fluttering may be felt by the patient when the arrhythmia produces a rapid heart rate.

Dizziness or lightheadedness: This is another symptom caused by the heart's inability to pump blood efficiently. The blood pressure may decrease during an arrhythmia causing these symptoms. This is more common in slow heart rates as in heart blocks.

Fainting: Severe arrhythmias can reduce blood flow to the brain, causing loss of consciousness. This can also be due to the lowered blood pressure during an arrhythmia. This is often seen in complete heart block.

Management

Medications: Drugs like beta-blockers, anti-arrhythmic drugs or blood thinners are used to control heart rate and prevent blood clots. The anti-arrhythmic drugs are those that control the arrhythmia and restore the normal rhythm of the heart. Blood thinners are given in some arrhythmias as the chances of blood clotting inside the heart or blood vessels is increased during the arrhythmias, especially AFib where the heart beat is irregular.

Defibrillation: In life-threatening cases, a quick shock to the heart using a defibrillator can restore a normal rhythm.

Pacemakers and Implantable Cardioverter-Defibrillators (**ICDs**): Doctors may use medication to help the heart beat more regularly. In more severe cases, they may need to insert a *Temporary Pacemaker*. This is a small device that sends gentle electrical signals to help the heart maintain a steady rhythm until a more permanent solution is in place. This pacemaker helps ensure that blood continues to flow properly through the body, preventing symptoms like dizziness or fainting caused by a very slow heartbeat. This is often needed in very slow heart rates as in complete heart block. Some patients may need a *Permanent Pacemaker* if the low heart rate persists even after recovering from the heart attack.

An *Implantable Cardioverter Defibrillator* (**ICD**) is a small device placed in the chest to monitor and correct dangerous heart rhythms. If the heart suddenly beats too fast or irregularly (*Ventricular Fibrillation*), the ICD gives a mild shock to restore a normal rhythm. It is usually implanted in patients after a heart attack if they have a high risk of life-threatening arrhythmias that could cause the heart to stop unexpectedly.

Lifestyle changes: Reducing caffeine, managing high blood pressure, and avoiding stress can often help prevent arrhythmias.

Cardiac Arrest

Sudden Cardiac Arrest (**SCA**) is a life-threatening condition where the heart abruptly stops functioning due to an irregular heart rhythm. This causes the heart to stop pumping blood to the rest of the body. When this happens, a person's breathing will stop, and they will quickly lose consciousness. Without immediate medical attention, cardiac arrest can lead to death within minutes.

Cardiac arrest occurs because the heart's electrical system, which controls the heartbeat, malfunctions. Normally, the heart beats in a regular, coordinated way to pump blood effectively. However, during cardiac arrest, this electrical system becomes chaotic, causing the heart to quiver instead of pumping blood effectively. One of the most common irregular rhythms that leads to cardiac arrest is called *Ventricular Fibrillation*, where the heart's ventricles (the main pumping chambers) start twitching erratically without contracting synchronously. As a result blood stops flowing to vital organs including the brain.

Asystole, often called "flatlining," is another cause of cardiac arrest when the heart completely stops beating and there is no electrical activity or movement. The heart is still. Here the ECG monitor shows a flat line instead of the normal graph. This means blood is no longer being pumped to the body, making it a life-threatening emergency. Immediate CPR and advanced medical care are needed to try to restart the heart.

> *David, a 50-year-old bank manager, was at the library with his 12-year-old son when he suddenly collapsed, clutching his chest in severe pain. Alarmed, the librarian rushed to his side and quickly realized David had suffered a sudden Cardiac Arrest. Unable to detect a pulse, the librarian, trained in Cardiopulmonary Resuscitation (CPR), immediately started performing chest compressions. Meanwhile, his assistant called for emergency services, and an ambulance was dispatched without delay.*
>
> *When the emergency medical team arrived, they found the librarian performing CPR. Upon assessment, they discovered David was in Ventricular Fibrillation, a life-threatening heart rhythm. The team immediately defibrillated him using a shock, which restored his heart to a normal rhythm. David was then rushed to the hospital, where a coronary angiography revealed a complete blockage in the left anterior descending coronary artery. A cardiologist performed an emergency angioplasty, placing a stent to restore blood flow.*
>
> *Thanks to the librarian's quick and timely action, David made a remarkable recovery, leaving the hospital a week later with minimal damage to his heart.*

Although sudden cardiac arrest can happen without warning due to many causes, it is often linked to a heart attack. A heart attack can interfere with the heart's electrical signals, leading to dangerous rhythms that can trigger a cardiac arrest. In fact, most cases of cardiac arrest are caused by heart attacks. *A heart attack is a problem with blood flow, while cardiac arrest is an issue with the heart's electrical system.*

Other factors can also contribute to cardiac arrest, such as low levels of essential minerals like potassium or magnesium, which are important for normal heart function. When these levels become too low or too high, it can disrupt the electrical signals in the heart and increase the risk of cardiac arrest.

Immediate treatment is crucial to save a person's life during cardiac arrest. Two key emergency treatments are Cardiopulmonary Resuscitation (**CPR**) and the use of an *Automated External Defibrillator* (**AED**). CPR involves chest compressions to manually pump blood through the body, while an AED delivers a controlled electric shock to the heart to restore a normal rhythm. Survival from cardiac arrest is possible, but only if these life-saving measures are applied quickly. For every minute without treatment, the chances of survival drop significantly.

With rapid and appropriate medical intervention, many people can recover from sudden cardiac arrest. However, quick action is essential to avoid permanent damage or death. *Cardiopulmonary resuscitation* is dealt with in detail in Chapter 24.

Cardiogenic Shock

Cardiogenic Shock is a life-threatening condition that happens when the heart is so severely damaged that it cannot pump enough blood to meet the body's needs, causing a severe drop in blood pressure. Cardiogenic shock usually occurs after a massive heart attack that destroys a large portion of the heart muscle. The heart becomes too weak to pump blood effectively, and as a result, vital organs like the brain, kidneys, and liver do not get enough oxygen.

Symptoms of cardiogenic shock

The main symptoms of cardiogenic shock are discussed below in brief.

Very low blood pressure: Following the heart attack, patients may feel extremely weak or faint because their blood pressure is dangerously low. The systolic blood pressure is below 90 mmHg.

Confusion or loss of consciousness: Lack of oxygen to the brain can cause mental confusion or fainting.

Cold, clammy skin: The body reduces blood flow to not so important structures in the body like the skin and extremities to protect vital organs like the brain, heart, kidneys and liver, causing the skin to feel cool and damp.

Rapid breathing: The body tries to compensate for the lack of oxygen by increasing the breathing rate. This fast rate of breathing makes the patient further drowsy.

Management.

Some of the important features of management of cardiogenic shock are discussed below.

Medications: Drugs named *Vasopressors* help raise blood pressure by tightening (*constricting*) blood vessels, while *Inotropic Agents* are those that strengthen the heart's contractions and thereby improve pumping.

Oxygen therapy: Additional oxygen is often given to ensure organs are getting enough oxygen.

Mechanical support: In severe cases, devices like an *Intra-Aortic Balloon Pump* (**IABP**) or a *Ventricular Assist Device* (**VAD**) may be used to help the heart pump more blood.

Surgery: If cardiogenic shock is caused by a blocked artery, emergency procedures like *Angioplasty* (to open the artery) or *Bypass Surgery* (to reroute blood flow) may be necessary.

Blood Clots

After a heart attack, patients are at higher risk of developing blood clots (*Thrombus*), which can lead to serious conditions such as strokes or *Pulmonary Embolism* (a clot within the arteries in the lungs).

After a heart attack, the body may try to repair damaged blood vessels, which can sometimes lead to clots forming in the bloodstream. Additionally, if patients are less active during recovery, blood flow slows down, increasing the risk of clots.

Blood clots can be of different types depending on the location where they form.

Vasu was a 60 year old security officer in a major company. He was slim and exercised regularly. He was careful with his diet. His only weakness was that he smoked about 20 – 25 cigarettes a day, especially during night duty to keep awake. One night, while he was on duty, smoking as usual, he felt a severe pain in his left arm followed by profuse sweating. Soon he collapsed. His colleague, who was on duty with him immediately summoned an ambulance and took him to a multispecialty hospital nearby where the doctors found him to have had a severe heart attack. His systolic blood pressure was very low at 70 mmHg, and he was confused and disoriented.

The doctors diagnosed a massive heart attack complicated by Cardiogenic Shock. The doctors started intravenous medications immediately and used other measures like an Intraaortic Balloon Pump to try to stabilize his condition. He had hardly any urine output. In spite of the valiant efforts of the doctors, Vasu had a sudden cardiac arrest due to ventricular fibrillation from which he could not be resuscitated despite efforts of the cardiac team for more than an hour. Vasu succumbed to the heart attack.

Deep vein thrombosis (**DVT**): A clot that forms in the deep veins of the legs, causing pain and swelling can occur especially if the patient is bedridden for long. If part of a blood clot breaks loose and travels to the heart, it moves through a large vein into the heart's right side and then to the lungs. Once in the lungs, a large clot can block a major blood vessel within the lungs, leading to a serious condition called a *Pulmonary Embolism*.

This blockage can severely affect blood flow in the lungs and requires urgent medical attention.

Pulmonary embolism (**PE**): A life-threatening condition that happens when a clot blocks blood flow in the lungs, leading to sudden shortness of breath and chest pain. This is often a clot that has dislodged from one of the clots in the deep leg veins and traveled up into the lungs to cause a PE.

Symptoms of blood clots

Pain or swelling in the leg may indicate deep vein thrombosis. Sudden shortness of breath or chest pain may be a sign of a pulmonary embolism.

Sudden weakness or confusion may occur if a clot blocks blood flow to the brain. One part of the body like a limb or one half of the body may become paralyzed (*Stroke*). Sometimes, the patient may be unable to speak, or speech may be slurred in case of a stroke.

Blood clots originating in the left ventricle of the heart after a heart attack can migrate along the blood stream to block various arteries in different parts of the body. Some of these sites where blood clots may lodge causing block are described briefly below.

Emboli

Emboli refer to blood clots that can form in the heart after a heart attack and travel through the bloodstream, blocking blood vessels elsewhere in the body. These blockages can cause severe complications, such as a *Stroke* (if the clot moves to the brain) or limb ischemia (if the clot blocks blood flow to the legs or arms). Emboli can severely damage organs by cutting off their blood supply and require quick intervention to prevent permanent damage or death.

Stroke

A stroke is a serious complication of a heart attack that occurs when a blood clot forms in the heart and travels to the brain, blocking blood flow. When part of the brain is deprived of oxygen and nutrients, brain cells begin to die, potentially causing paralysis, speech difficulties, and cognitive impairments. A stroke is a medical emergency, and quick treatment can improve the chances of recovery and reduce the risk of long-term damage.

Limb Ischemia

Limb *ischemia* (deprival of blood supply) occurs when the blood supply to the arms or legs is severely reduced or blocked after a heart attack, often due to a clot. Without proper blood flow, the tissue in the affected limb (a toe or part of the foot) may 'die' and this tissue death is called *Gangrene*. Ischemia of the limb causes pain and numbness, and, in severe cases, tissue death (*gangrene*). This condition may need *amputation* (surgical removal) of the limb or part of the limb. Immediate treatment is crucial to restore blood flow and prevent permanent damage. Once gangrene occurs, that part may have to be surgically removed.

Renal Infarction

Renal infarction is a complication where a blood clot blocks the blood supply to the kidneys, causing kidney tissue to die. This can result in sharp pain in flank and abdomen, nausea, and reduced kidney function. Blood may be present in urine. In severe cases, it can lead to kidney failure, where the kidneys are no longer able to filter waste from the blood effectively. This condition requires prompt medical treatment to prevent long-term damage to the kidneys and other organs.

Mesenteric Ischemia

Mesenteric ischemia occurs when the blood flow to the intestines is blocked, usually by a clot that has traveled from the heart after a heart attack. This condition causes severe abdominal pain, especially after eating, and can lead to intestinal damage or tissue death (*gangrene*) if left untreated. Mesenteric ischemia is a serious, life-threatening condition that requires emergency surgery to restore blood flow and prevent irreversible damage to the intestines.

Management.

Blood clots are managed depending on their location and severity of symptoms.

Blood thinners: Drugs like *Heparin* or *Warfarin* are used to prevent clots from forming or growing. These medications are taken long-term to reduce the risk of future clots.

Compression stockings: Special stockings that improve circulation in the legs, helping prevent clots. For patients who are bedridden, inflatable stockings are available. These inflate at regular intervals to function as a peripheral pump to pump blood from the legs back to the heart.

Physical activity: Gentle movement, as recommended by doctors, can help keep blood flowing and reduce the risk of clots. Bedridden patients should move their feet and legs frequently to aid blood circulation in the lower limbs.

Surgery or procedures: In severe cases, doctors may perform a *Thrombectomy* (surgical removal of the clot) or insert a *"Vena Cava filter"* in the inferior vena cava, which catches clots before they can travel to the lungs from the veins in the legs.

The important aspect of management of blood clots is to prevent their formation, especially in the deep veins of the legs. This is achieved by moving the limbs and using compression stockings and other measures is the patient is bed ridden.

Ischemic Cardiomyopathy (ICM)

Ischemic Cardiomyopathy is a condition where the heart muscle weakens due to insufficient blood flow, often after a heart attack. The word '*cardiomyopathy*' indicates 'disease of the heart muscle'. This weakens the heart's ability to pump blood efficiently. Over time, this can lead to congestive heart failure (**CHF**), where the heart cannot keep up with the body's needs. This results in symptoms like swelling (*edema*), fatigue, shortness of breath, and fluid buildup in the lungs and other parts of the body. The symptoms and signs are the same as those of congestive heart failure.

Pericardial Effusion

Pericardial effusion is the abnormal accumulation of fluid in the sac around the heart (*pericardium*). The pericardium is thin sac that surrounds the heart and helps support it. It has two layers - an outer and inner layer, with a little bit of fluid between these layers. After a heart attack, the pericardium around the heart may become inflamed, leading to fluid buildup. This inflammation of the pericardium is called *Pericarditis*.

Sometimes fluid accumulates between these layers of the pericardium (*Pericardial Effusion*). If too much fluid accumulates, it can compress the heart, limiting its ability to pump blood effectively. This condition, called *Cardiac Tamponade*, can be life-threatening if not treated promptly. Immediately draining the excess fluid can relieve the pressure and allow the heart to function normally again. Pericardial effusion and cardiac tamponade can be easily diagnosed by echocardiography.

Management of Complications

Managing the complications that arise after a heart attack is a multifaceted process, requiring a combination of immediate medical treatments, long-term medications, lifestyle changes, and ongoing care. Occasionally the help of a surgeon is needed to manage certain complications. Each part of this management strategy is designed to support the heart, prevent further damage, and help patients live healthier lives.

Medical Interventions

In the first stage of managing heart attack complications, doctors focus on stabilizing the patient and addressing any immediate threats to health and life. The goal is to restore normal heart function and prevent additional damage.

Medications

Medications are crucial in managing heart attack complications. Different types of drugs work together to stabilize the heart, prevent clots, and control symptoms:

Blood thinners, Diuretics, Beta blockers and ACE inhibitors are given to patients after a heart attack when there are complications. Aspirin or clopidogrel help reduce the risk of blood clots forming in the arteries. This is important because clots can block blood flow and cause another heart attack or stroke. Diuretics help reduce fluid buildup in the body, especially for patients with heart failure. By removing excess fluid, diuretics ease the workload on the heart and reduce symptoms like swelling and shortness of breath. Beta-blockers slow down the heart rate and lower blood pressure, reducing the heart's demand for oxygen. This helps prevent further damage to the heart muscle, especially in people who have had a heart attack. ACE inhibitors help relax blood vessels and lower blood pressure, making it easier for the heart to pump blood. This is important for people with weakened hearts, as it helps prevent heart failure from worsening.

Surgery or procedures

In some cases, medications alone are not enough to manage complications, and more advanced medical procedures may be necessary:

Angioplasty used to reopen blocked arteries helps in restoring the blood circulation to the heart muscle.

Pacemakers or defibrillators are used when there is an arrhythmia. An *implanted defibrillator* can detect dangerous rhythms, like ventricular fibrillation, and deliver a shock automatically to restore a normal heartbeat. This can be implanted on to the chest of the patient under the skin.

Once the immediate complications have been addressed, long-term care is essential to prevent further heart problems and help the patient recover fully.

Cardiac rehabilitation

One of the most important parts of ongoing care after a heart attack is cardiac rehabilitation. This is a structured program that helps patients rebuild their strength and improve their heart health. It usually includes Supervised exercise, Education of the patient and Emotional support for the patient. For more details refer to Chapter 18 on *Cardiac Rehabilitation*.

Lifestyle changes

Long-term heart health depends heavily on making certain lifestyle changes. These changes not only help prevent complications but also promote overall well-being. The lifestyle changes have been described in detail in the Chapter 20 on *Prevention of Heart Attack*.

Regular Monitoring

After a heart attack, patients require ongoing medical supervision to monitor their progress and adjust treatments as needed. Regular follow-ups with healthcare providers are a key part of this process.

Regular check-ups with a cardiologist help monitor how well the heart is recovering. During these visits, doctors may perform tests, review medications, and make any necessary changes to the treatment plan.

High blood pressure and cholesterol are major risk factors for heart disease. Patients will need regular tests to ensure these levels are within a healthy range. If necessary, adjustments to diet, lifestyle, or medications will be made to keep these levels under control.

In some cases, doctors may recommend tests like echocardiograms or stress tests to evaluate how well the heart is functioning. These tests help detect any new or worsening issues with heart function.

Patients are encouraged to pay close attention to any symptoms, such as chest pain, shortness of breath, or swelling in the legs. If these symptoms occur, they should seek medical advice promptly to prevent further complications.

Managing heart attack complications is an ongoing process that involves immediate medical treatments, long-term care, and consistent monitoring. Medications and procedures help address immediate issues, while cardiac rehabilitation and lifestyle changes build the foundation for long-term heart health. Regular follow-ups ensure that the patient's recovery is on track and that any potential problems are caught early.

Key Takeaways

- *Heart attacks can lead to serious complications, including damage to the heart and other vital organs.*
- *Acute pulmonary edema occurs when fluid accumulates in the lungs, leading to breathing difficulties and reduced oxygen supply, often*

requiring urgent treatment such as diuretics or mechanical ventilation.
- Heart failure may develop when the heart's ability to pump blood is compromised, needing long-term management with medications, lifestyle changes, or surgical interventions.
- Arrhythmias, or irregular heartbeats, are common after a heart attack and can range from mild to life-threatening, often treated with medications, pacemakers, or defibrillators.
- Mechanical complications like ventricular aneurysm involve structural damage to the heart muscle, potentially requiring surgical repair to prevent rupture.
- Cardiogenic shock, a critical condition where the heart cannot supply enough blood to the body, may require aggressive treatments like inotropes, vasopressors, or mechanical support devices.
- Blood clots can form in the heart after a heart attack, leading to emboli that may cause stroke or block arteries in other parts of the body, often managed with anticoagulants.
- Stroke and peripheral artery embolism are serious complications resulting from clots, requiring prompt treatment with thrombolytics, anticoagulation, or surgical intervention.
- Each complication requires a tailored management approach, often combining medications, interventions, and lifestyle changes to improve patient outcomes.

Chapter 17 CONVALESCENCE AFTER HEART ATTACK

Convalescence after a heart attack is a critical phase in the recovery journey, requiring time, patience, and proactive care. This chapter focuses on the gradual healing process that follows a heart attack, offering guidance on how to manage the physical and emotional aspects of recovery. Patients often face new challenges after leaving the hospital, such as adjusting to medications, incorporating lifestyle changes, and participating in cardiac rehabilitation. Knowing the importance of rest, light physical activity, and regular medical follow-ups can help prevent further complications and support the healing process. In this chapter, you will also find insights into how diet, exercise, and stress management play vital roles in protecting the heart.

Convalescence means the gradual healing (through rest) after any sickness or injury. Recovery after a heart attack is not something that happens overnight. It is a gradual process that takes time, care, and commitment. This period of recovery, known as convalescence, is critical for healing the heart, regaining strength, and preventing future heart issues. While it may seem daunting at first, understanding the recovery process and taking proactive steps can help you return to a healthy and fulfilling life.

This and the next couple of chapters have many features in common. It may seem that many of the details are repeated. However, they address different aspects of the recovery process after a heart attack and its preventive aspects. The reader is requested to read these chapters to acquire a comprehensive knowledge of the recovery process.

The Recovery Process

Once you are discharged from the hospital, the real work of recovery begins. Your body and heart need time to heal, and you will need to make certain adjustments to your lifestyle. The recovery period is crucial for ensuring that the damage caused by the heart attack does not lead to further complications.

After leaving the hospital, you will need to attend regular follow-up appointments with your doctor or cardiologist. These visits are essential for monitoring your heart's health, checking for any complications, and adjusting medications if necessary. Regular check-ups also help ensure that you are progressing well and staying on track with your recovery plan. You will continue to take medications that were prescribed during your hospital stay. The medications which the doctors prescribe on discharge have already been discussed previously.

Other drugs may be prescribed depending on the need. Taking these medications exactly as prescribed is key to preventing further heart issues and promoting recovery.

Your heart has been through a major event, and it needs time to heal. It is normal to feel more tired or weaker than usual in the early days of recovery. Rest is important, but so is staying active—your doctor will guide you on when and how to start introducing light physical activities back into your routine.

Post-discharge care
Cardiac rehabilitation

One of the most effective ways to speed up recovery and regain strength is through cardiac rehabilitation. This program is usually tailored to your specific needs and includes:

<u>Supervised exercise</u>: Gentle physical activities are carefully monitored by healthcare professionals to help your heart regain strength without over exertion.

<u>Education on heart health</u>: Lifestyle changes that can improve heart health, such as dietary adjustments and managing stress are also taught to the patients.

Emotional support: Recovering from a heart attack can be emotionally challenging, with many people experiencing anxiety or fear about their heart's condition. Cardiac rehabilitation offers counseling and support to help you manage these feelings and build confidence as you recover.

After a heart attack, a cardiac rehabilitation program can help rebuild strength and improve heart health. A typical program involves the following aspects.

- A person should always consult a doctor before beginning any new exercise program after a heart attack. In a rehabilitation program the doctor guides the exercise program.
- Low-impact aerobic exercises like walking, cycling on a stationary bike, using an elliptical machine, and rowing are commonly included. Some programs may also add water aerobics or light strength training with weights or resistance bands.
- Exercises start with low intensity and gradually increase as the individual gets stronger. Sessions always include warm-up and cool-down periods to prepare the body and prevent injury.
- During each session, healthcare professionals carefully track heart rate, blood pressure, and other vital signs to ensure safety and avoid strain on the heart.
- The exercises are tailored to each person's fitness level and specific needs, adjusting over time to support progress.
- The patient is told to stop exercising and seek medical help if he feel chest pain, dizziness, shortness of breath, or other unusual symptoms.

- Regular exercise is essential for maintaining heart health and can support recovery and overall well-being. Being consistent is the hallmark of a good cardiac rehabilitation program.

With guidance and gradual progress, these exercises can help make a positive impact on heart health and recovery. Cardiac rehabilitation is a key part of the recovery process and greatly improves your chances of returning to a healthy and active life.

Typical recovery timeline

Recovering from a heart attack is different for everyone. How long it takes to feel "normal" again depends on several factors, including the severity of the heart attack, your overall health, your associated conditions and how well you follow your recovery plan. Patience is important during this time, as your body heals at its own pace.

<u>First few days to weeks</u>: In the initial phase of recovery, it is common to feel fatigued, weak, and low on energy. Even simple tasks like walking short distances or climbing stairs may feel exhausting. You may also experience soreness or discomfort, especially in the chest area. Rest is important during this period, but doctors will also encourage light activity, such as short walks, to keep your circulation moving and help prevent complications like blood clots in the leg veins. One should not get disheartened by the initial weakness.

<u>First month</u>: After a few weeks, many patients start to feel stronger, especially if they are participating in a cardiac rehabilitation program. Light activities such as walking around the house or doing simple household

chores may become easier, but more strenuous activities, such as heavy lifting or intense exercise, are still restricted.

Three to six months: By this stage, most people begin to feel much more like themselves. Energy levels improve significantly, and many can return to regular activities, including work or hobbies. Patients who follow their recovery plan closely and participate in cardiac rehabilitation often report feeling stronger and more confident with time.

When to expect full recovery

Physical recovery: For most people, it takes several months to fully recover from a heart attack. While some may regain their strength within three to six months, others may need up to a year depending on their condition. The severity of the heart attack and the occurrence of complications like heart failure, plays a significant role in how quickly a person can recover physically. Recovery takes longer in those with complications.

Emotional recovery: Recovering emotionally from a heart attack can take even longer than physical recovery. It is common to feel anxious about the possibility of having another heart attack, and some people may struggle with fear or depression. Addressing emotional recovery is just as important as physical healing, and counseling or support groups can be helpful during this time.

Factors affecting speed of recovery

<u>Severity of the heart attack</u>: People who had a mild heart attack tend to recover faster than those who experienced severe heart damage.

<u>Age and overall health</u>: Older individuals or those with existing health conditions, such as high blood pressure, diabetes, kidney disease, chronic lung disease or obesity, may have a slower recovery process.

<u>Adherence to the recovery plan</u>: Patients who diligently follow their doctor's recommendations on medications, diet, and lifestyle changes tend to recover more quickly and have fewer complications. Sticking to your recovery plan is essential for ensuring that your heart heals properly.

Recovering from a heart attack is a journey that requires patience, commitment, and careful attention to your health. The first few days and weeks after leaving the hospital are critical for healing, and ongoing care, including cardiac rehabilitation and lifestyle changes, plays a key role in helping you regain strength and prevent future heart issues. While the timeline for feeling normal again varies from person to person, following the recovery plan and attending regular follow-up appointments with the doctor will help the patient stay on track. By taking control of your recovery and making the necessary changes to the lifestyle, a person can reduce the risk of future heart problems and enjoy a healthier, more active life.

Changes in Lifestyle

A heart attack often marks a turning point in a person's life. It is a serious event that signals the need for long-term lifestyle changes to support heart health and prevent future problems. Once recovery begins, patients must make adjustments to their daily routine, including their physical activity, diet, and how they manage stress. These changes are vital for healing and for reducing the risk of another heart attack.

Physical Activity

Getting active again is one of the most important parts of recovery, but it must be done carefully to avoid putting too much strain on the heart. Regular physical activity helps the heart get stronger over time, but it should be introduced gradually, especially after a heart attack. Those who join a cardiac rehabilitation program are taught how to return to normal life. Others need to follow certain principles.

<u>Starting slow</u>: It is important for patients to start with light physical activities, such as short, gentle walks. Initially, these walks should only last a few minutes, but as the heart gets stronger, patients can gradually increase both the duration and intensity of exercise. The key is to go at a comfortable pace and listen to the body's signals.

<u>Supervised exercise</u>: Cardiac rehabilitation programs are designed to help patients exercise safely under the supervision of medical professionals. These programs guide patients through appropriate levels of physical activity and monitor their progress to ensure the heart is not overworked. Participating in a supervised program builds confidence and ensures that patients are exercising at a level that is safe for them.

Types of Exercise

Aerobic exercises are activities like walking, cycling, or swimming, and are excellent for heart health. Aerobic exercise helps improve circulation, strengthens the heart muscle, and lowers blood pressure. These activities should be done regularly, but it is important to start slowly and build up endurance over time.

Strength training are exercises to be undertaken after receiving approval from a doctor. Patients can begin light strength training using resistance bands or lifting light weights. These can help rebuild muscle strength, which may have weakened during the recovery period. Strength training also supports overall fitness and helps with daily activities.

Regular physical activity is essential for managing heart health after a heart attack. Exercise helps lower blood pressure, reduce cholesterol levels, and control body weight—three factors that are critical for preventing another heart attack. Additionally, staying active improves mood and increases energy, which can make a big difference in the recovery process.

Diet

Diet plays a central role in heart health, particularly after a heart attack. The foods you eat can either support your recovery or contribute to further heart problems. A heart-healthy diet focuses on reducing foods that clog the arteries and increasing foods that nourish the heart.

Foods that are high in unhealthy fats, such as red meat, butter, and full-fat dairy products, contribute to plaque buildup in the arteries. This plaque can block blood flow to the heart, increasing the risk of another heart attack. Reducing these foods helps protect the arteries and keeps blood flowing smoothly.

Fresh fruits, vegetables, and whole grains are rich in fiber, vitamins, and minerals that support heart health. These foods help lower cholesterol levels and provide the nutrients needed for overall well-being. Making plant-based foods the foundation of the diet is a simple and effective way to improve heart health.

Too much salt raises blood pressure, which puts extra strain on the heart. To keep blood pressure under control, it is important to limit salt. This means cutting back on processed foods, which often contain hidden sodium, and avoiding adding extra salt to meals.

Heart-Healthy Eating Habits

Mediterranean diet: A diet that emphasizes fruits, vegetables, whole grains, lean proteins (like fish), and healthy fats (like olive oil) is widely recommended for heart health. This eating pattern has been shown to reduce the risk of heart attacks and other cardiovascular problems. (**Fig. 17.1**).

Portion control: Eating smaller, more frequent meals throughout the day can help prevent overeating and maintain a healthy weight. Managing portion sizes is important for weight control, which is a key factor in reducing the risk of heart disease.

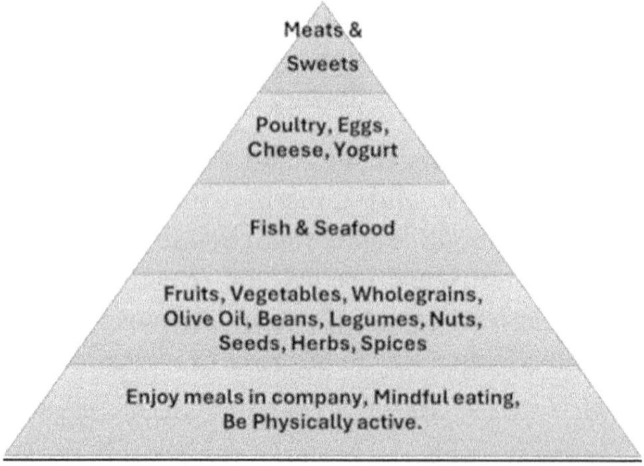

```
              Meats &
              Sweets

          Poultry, Eggs,
          Cheese, Yogurt

           Fish & Seafood

     Fruits, Vegetables, Wholegrains,
     Olive Oil, Beans, Legumes, Nuts,
          Seeds, Herbs, Spices

   Enjoy meals in company, Mindful eating,
          Be Physically active.
```

Fig. 17. 1. The Mediterranean Diet

At the base of the triangle, the focus is on mindful eating and enjoying meals in the company of others. The next tier emphasizes a plant-based foundation with plenty of fruits, vegetables, grains, and nuts. Moving upward, fish and seafood are highlighted as key components to include regularly for healthy fats. The fourth tier suggests moderate consumption of poultry, eggs, cheese, and yogurt. At the apex, meat and sweets are to be eaten sparingly, rounding out a balanced and healthful Mediterranean approach.

(Image Courtesy of the author from the book "Diabetes Demystified")

In addition to physical activity and diet, recovering from a heart attack requires adjustments to everyday routines. Managing stress and avoiding unhealthy habits are important for long-term heart health.

Managing Stress

Stress is a significant risk factor for heart disease. It causes the body to release hormones that can raise blood pressure and strain the heart. Relaxation practices, such as deep breathing exercises, meditation, or yoga, help reduce stress and promote a sense of calm. These techniques are simple but effective ways to protect the heart from the negative effects of stress.

Returning to Work

Returning to work after a heart attack depends on the severity of the heart attack and the type of job. Many people can return to desk jobs or light duties within a few weeks to a few months. However, those with more physically demanding jobs may need to wait longer or adjust their workload to avoid putting too much pressure on the heart. It is important to consult with one's doctor about when and how to return to work.

Avoiding Smoking and Alcohol

Smoking is one of the leading risk factors for heart attacks. The chemicals in cigarettes damage the blood vessels, raise blood pressure, and increase the risk of blood clots. For patients who smoke, quitting is one of the most important steps they can take to protect their heart. Smoking cessation programs and resources can help patients quit for good.

While moderate alcohol consumption may be allowed for some patients, it is important to limit intake to avoid putting extra strain on the heart. Drinking too much alcohol can raise blood pressure and contribute to other heart-related problems, so it is best to stick to the doctor's guidelines regarding alcohol. Alcohol also contain empty calories which tends to increase the weight of the person.

Emotional Recovery

Recovering from a heart attack is not just about physical healing—it also involves addressing emotional challenges. Many people experience anxiety, depression, or a sense of fear after a heart attack. It is important to recognize these feelings and seek help if needed.

Anxiety

It is normal to feel anxious after a heart attack, especially about the possibility of having another one. Patients may also worry about their physical limitations and whether they will be able to return to their normal activities.

Talking to a therapist or counselor can help patients manage their anxiety. *Cognitive-behavioral therapy* (**CBT**) and other forms of counseling can provide tools to manage fears and develop a positive mindset. Participating in a cardiac rehabilitation support group can also be beneficial, as patients share their experiences and encourage each other through recovery.

Depression

Depression is not uncommon after a heart attack. Patients may feel a loss of interest in activities they once enjoyed or experience feelings of sadness and hopelessness. These feelings can make it harder to stay motivated during recovery.

Treating depression after a heart attack is crucial because it can negatively impact recovery, reduce adherence to medical advice, and increase the risk of further heart complications. Patients with post-heart attack depression are at a higher risk for future cardiac events and mortality. Studies show that individuals with depression after a heart attack have up to a 2-3 times higher risk of death compared to those without depression, underscoring the importance of prompt mental health care.

If feelings of depression persist, it is important to talk to a doctor or mental health professional. Therapy or medications may be recommended to help manage symptoms. Staying engaged in cardiac rehabilitation and staying active can also improve mood and overall mental health.

In conclusion, recovering from a heart attack involves making significant changes to physical activity, diet, and daily routines. Additionally, emotional recovery is just as important as physical healing. By adopting a heart-healthy lifestyle, patients can regain their strength and reduce their risk of future heart attacks, leading to a healthier, more active life.

Key Takeaways

- *Recovery after a heart attack is a gradual process that requires time, rest, and dedication to regain strength and improve heart health.*
- *Regular follow-up appointments with healthcare providers are crucial for monitoring heart health,*

adjusting medications, and ensuring recovery is on track.
- *Medications such as blood thinners, beta-blockers, and statins are prescribed to support heart recovery and prevent further complications.*
- *Rest is essential, but light physical activity, guided by medical advice, is also important for promoting circulation and preventing complications.*
- *Cardiac rehabilitation programs provide supervised exercise, heart health education, and emotional support, helping patients regain strength and confidence.*
- *The recovery timeline varies for each individual, but patience and adherence to the recovery plan are key to long-term health improvements.*
- *Emotional recovery may take longer than physical recovery; addressing anxiety or depression is an important aspect of healing.*
- *Lifestyle changes, including adjustments to diet, physical activity, and stress management, are essential for supporting heart health during convalescence.*
- *The severity of the heart attack, age, and overall health significantly impact the speed and ease of recovery.*
- *Participation in cardiac rehabilitation, combined with proper medication adherence and lifestyle changes, greatly enhances the chances of a full and healthy recovery.*

Chapter 18 CARDIAC REHABILITATION

After surviving a heart attack, ongoing care and rehabilitation are essential to promote healing, prevent future issues, and improve long-term health. Post-heart attack care involves taking prescribed medications, attending follow-up appointments, and undergoing tests to monitor heart function. Medications such as aspirin, beta-blockers, and statins help manage blood pressure, cholesterol, and prevent further damage. Equally important is patient education, which empowers individuals to manage symptoms, medications, and make necessary lifestyle changes. Cardiac rehabilitation complements this by offering a structured, medically supervised program focusing on exercise, nutrition, and risk management.

Recovering from a heart attack is an ongoing journey, requiring a combination of medical care, lifestyle changes, and emotional support. Post-heart attack care and rehabilitation are essential in helping patients heal, reduce the risk of future heart problems, and lead healthier lives. This comprehensive chapter explains the key components of recovery, including cardiac rehabilitation, medication management, and the importance of follow-up care.

After surviving a heart attack, the journey to recovery is ongoing. Key aspects of care include taking medications, attending follow-up appointments, and undergoing tests to monitor heart health. These measures support the heart's recovery and help reduce the risk of future heart issues.

What is Cardiac Rehabilitation?

Cardiac rehabilitation is a structured program aimed at improving the health and well-being of patients who have experienced serious heart issues. It combines exercise, education, and support to guide patients through recovery and help them make long-lasting lifestyle changes that support heart health.

The main goal of cardiac rehabilitation is to help patients recover from heart-related events or surgeries by improving physical fitness, promoting healthier habits, and reducing the likelihood of future heart problems. It is a comprehensive program that focuses on strengthening the heart and improving the overall quality of life.

Cardiac rehabilitation is highly recommended for anyone who has had a heart attack, heart surgery (like a bypass or valve surgery), angina, or a heart procedure such as angioplasty or stent placement. It is also beneficial for those with other heart conditions or those at high risk of heart disease.

Cardiac rehabilitation typically begins while the patient is still in the hospital and continues as an outpatient service once they are discharged. Each program is personalized to meet the individual needs of the patient, taking into account their heart condition, fitness level, and overall health. The program usually includes a combination of supervised exercise, nutritional counseling, and emotional support.

Long-Term Benefits

Research has shown that patients who complete a cardiac rehabilitation program enjoy better long-term outcomes. These benefits include a significantly lower risk of having another heart attack and, in many cases, a longer life expectancy.

By managing risk factors, forming healthy habits, and sticking to medication, patients are far less likely to suffer another heart attack. Completing cardiac rehabilitation gives patients the tools and confidence to lead a healthier, more active life. They feel better equipped to manage their condition and prevent future heart problems. Cardiac rehabilitation provides the knowledge and support necessary to protect heart health and prevent further heart events.

Key components of Cardiac Rehabilitation

The three main elements of cardiac rehabilitation are Physical exercise, Nutrition and Lifestyle counseling, and emotional support. These components work together to help patients recover and prevent future heart problems. Cardiac rehabilitation focuses on lifestyle changes that significantly improve heart health and lower the risk of future heart problems.

1. Physical Exercise

Exercise is one of the most vital components of cardiac rehabilitation. Regular physical activity strengthens the heart, improves circulation, and boosts overall fitness.

In cardiac rehabilitation, exercise is carefully supervised by medical professionals. Patients are guided through activities that are safe for their heart condition, and the level of activity is gradually increased as the heart becomes stronger. This reduces the risk of overexertion and helps patients build confidence in their physical abilities.

The various types of exercises described previously are employed during cardiac rehabilitation. Aerobic activities like walking on a treadmill, cycling on a stationary bike, or swimming are commonly used in rehabilitation. These exercises improve cardiovascular endurance by helping the heart pump more efficiently and increasing blood flow throughout the body.

Strength training exercises are light resistance exercises, such as lifting small weights or using resistance bands, which help build muscle strength. This is especially important for patients who may have lost muscle mass due to prolonged illness or inactivity.

Regular exercise has many benefits for heart health. It lowers blood pressure, reduces cholesterol levels, helps control blood sugar, and assists with weight management—all of which are critical for preventing future heart attacks. Exercise also strengthens the heart, making it more resilient and better able to handle physical activity in the future. These are discussed in more detail in the next chapter 19 on *Lifestyle Changes After Heart Attack*.

2. Nutrition Counseling

Healthy eating is crucial for heart recovery, and nutrition counseling is a key part of cardiac rehabilitation. Patients learn how to make dietary changes that support heart health and prevent further damage to their cardiovascular system.

In cardiac rehabilitation, patients work with dietitians to create personalized meal plans that focus on heart-healthy foods. The goal is to reduce the intake of foods that contribute to clogged arteries such as foods high in unhealthy fats and sugars and increase nutrient-rich foods that support heart health.

Key elements of a heart-healthy diet

Limiting saturated and trans fats, reducing sodium (salt), increasing fruits, vegetables, and whole grains and moderating portion sizes are the most important aspects of a heart-healthy diet. Adopting a heart-healthy diet can significantly reduce the risk of future heart attacks and other cardiovascular problems. Eating well helps control weight, lower cholesterol, and keep blood pressure in check—factors that are all crucial for long-term heart health. This is discussed more elaborately in the next chapter 19 on *Lifestyle Changes After Heart Attack*.

3. Education About Heart Health

Education is another vital part of cardiac rehabilitation. Patients are taught about their heart condition and given the tools they need to manage their health effectively.

Topics covered

Patients learn about their specific heart condition, including what caused it and how to prevent future issues. For example, they learn about the role of blood pressure, cholesterol, and blood sugar in heart disease. They are also educated on how to recognize the warning signs of another heart attack, such as chest pain, shortness of breath, or sudden dizziness, so they can seek help quickly if necessary.

Practical tips

The program offers practical tips on making heart-healthy choices in daily life. Patients learn how to read food labels, prepare low-fat meals, and incorporate physical activity into their routines. They also receive guidance on important lifestyle changes like quitting smoking and limiting alcohol consumption, both of which are essential for heart health.

Long-term impact

Understanding heart health empowers patients to take control of their recovery and make informed decisions that improve their well-being. The education provided in cardiac rehabilitation helps patients manage their risk factors, stay on top of medications, and maintain a heart-healthy lifestyle for the long term.

Cardiac rehabilitation is a vital part of recovery after a heart attack or heart surgery. Through exercise, nutrition counseling, and education, it helps patients regain strength, reduce the risk of future heart problems, and take control of their health. This medically supervised program not only improves physical fitness but also offers emotional support and practical tools for long-term heart health. By participating in cardiac rehabilitation, patients can make positive lifestyle changes that lead to a healthier, more active life.

Recovering from a heart attack is about more than just surviving the immediate event. It involves adopting long-term changes that can protect your heart from future problems. This is where cardiac rehabilitation plays a crucial role. Cardiac rehabilitation is a comprehensive program designed not only to help people recover from a heart attack but also to prevent further heart complications. It achieves this by focusing on managing key risk factors and promoting healthy lifestyle habits.

Risk Factor Management

Heart attacks often occur due to certain risk factors like high blood pressure, high cholesterol, obesity, and diabetes. These conditions place extra strain on the heart and increase the likelihood of future heart issues if left untreated. Cardiac rehabilitation helps patients take control of these risks by offering guidance and support in managing them effectively.

One of the primary goals of cardiac rehabilitation is to control risk factors that can lead to another heart attack. For instance, high blood pressure forces the heart to work harder to pump blood, which weakens the heart over time. Rehabilitation programs teach patients how to manage their blood pressure through diet, exercise, and sometimes medication.

Carrying excess weight, especially around the abdomen, increases the burden on the heart. Many heart attack survivors are overweight, which further elevates their risk of future heart problems. Through cardiac rehabilitation, patients are provided with personalized diet and exercise plans to help them achieve a healthy weight. Even modest weight loss can significantly reduce stress on the heart and improve overall health.

Managing these factors effectively reduces the risk of another heart attack, giving patients a better chance of leading a long, healthy life.

Building Healthy Habits

A key component of cardiac rehabilitation is helping patients develop healthy habits that they can maintain for life. Often, lifestyle changes are what make the difference between a one-time heart attack and a recurring heart problem. The rehabilitation program does not just offer short-term solutions; it teaches people how to adopt a heart-healthy lifestyle that sticks.

Forming these habits helps protect the heart from further damage and significantly lowers the risk of recurring heart issues.

Psychological Support and Group Therapy

Recovering from a heart attack is not just about the physical healing process—your mental and emotional well-being is equally important. A heart attack can be a deeply traumatic experience, leaving many people feeling anxious, fearful, or even depressed about their future health. Cardiac rehabilitation recognizes this and includes psychological support and group therapy as critical components of recovery.

The Emotional Impact of a Heart Attack

Having a heart attack can trigger intense emotions. Many survivors find themselves overwhelmed by feelings of vulnerability or fear, while others may struggle with sadness or frustration.

It is common for patients to worry about having another heart attack, leading to constant anxiety. Some may also feel depressed due to changes in their health or lifestyle, or because they can no longer engage in activities they used to enjoy.

Mental health is a key part of recovery. Negative emotions like stress, anxiety, and depression can impact heart health by raising blood pressure and increasing heart rate, making it harder for the heart to recover. These feelings can also lead to unhealthy behaviors, like overeating, smoking, or avoiding exercise.

By addressing the emotional toll of a heart attack, cardiac rehabilitation helps patients achieve full recovery—both physically and mentally.

Psychological Support and Counseling

Cardiac rehabilitation includes counseling services designed to help patients cope with the emotional challenges of recovery. This can include one-on-one sessions with a counselor or psychologist, as well as teaching stress-reduction techniques.

In private sessions, patients have the opportunity to discuss their fears, anxieties, and emotional difficulties. Trained professionals help them develop coping strategies that make it easier to deal with these challenges.

Patients are also taught practical ways to manage stress, such as deep breathing exercises, meditation, or *Progressive Muscle Relaxation*. These techniques help reduce anxiety and promote emotional balance.

Group Therapy

Another vital aspect of emotional recovery is group therapy, where patients can share their experiences and find support from others who have gone through similar situations.

Many patients form lasting friendships with their peers in cardiac rehabilitation. These connections can continue to provide emotional support even after the formal program has ended, helping individuals stay motivated in their recovery

Cardiac rehabilitation thus, is a holistic program that addresses both the physical and emotional aspects of recovering from a heart attack. It equips patients with the tools to manage their risk factors, build healthy habits, and follow their medication plans, significantly reducing the risk of future heart problems. Equally important, cardiac rehabilitation provides crucial psychological support, helping patients deal with the emotional impact of their heart attack and offering opportunities for group therapy and peer connection.

> *Chandran, a 50-year-old chief carpenter in a large furniture manufacturing factory, led a team of fifty carpenters under constant pressure to meet strict deadlines. One day at work, he experienced severe chest pain and collapsed, leading to an urgent hospitalization where doctors diagnosed a heart attack. Immediate Coronary Angioplasty saved his life, but he was found to have a persistent Complete Heart Block, resulting in a dangerously low heart rate of 30 bpm. To stabilize his condition, doctors implanted a Permanent Pacemaker.*
>
> *Following his discharge, Chandran remained physically weak and emotionally distressed, as he was the primary provider for his family of five. Recognizing his dedication, the factory owner generously enrolled him in a Cardiac Rehabilitation program. Chandran participated in graded exercises, received dietary and medication guidance, and attended cognitive behavioral therapy to help him quit his long-standing smoking habit and address his depression.*
>
> *Three months later, Chandran had made a remarkable recovery. He returned to work, supervising his team with renewed energy, having lost ten pounds and embracing a smoking-free, active lifestyle. Chandran's cheerful disposition returned, and he felt fit and ready to resume his responsibilities in the factory.*

By combining these elements, cardiac rehab becomes a vital step toward both physical and emotional healing, helping patients lead healthier, longer lives.

Post-Heart Attack Medications

After a heart attack, doctors often prescribe medications to manage conditions like high cholesterol or to reduce the thickness of blood to prevent clots. However, many people struggle to follow their medication regimen consistently, either because they do not understand its importance, or they forget. Cardiac rehabilitation addresses this challenge by educating patients about the role of medications in heart health.

Patients are taught about the purpose of each prescribed medication, whether it is to lower cholesterol, control blood pressure, or prevent blood clots. Knowing how the medications work makes patients more likely to stick to their treatment plan.

Consistency in taking medications is key to preventing future heart problems. Cardiac rehabilitation emphasizes the importance of taking medications exactly as prescribed to avoid complications. Patients are encouraged to ask questions and seek help if they experience side effects or have trouble remembering to take their medications.

Medications play a crucial role in post-heart attack care. These drugs help the heart recover, reduce the risk of another heart attack, and manage underlying conditions like high blood pressure or high cholesterol. After a heart attack, several medications may be prescribed, and it is important to take them exactly as directed by your doctor.

Though medications after a heart attack have been discussed in previous chapters, they are discussed in a bit more detail here including their effects and side effects.

Aspirin

Aspirin is one of the most common medications prescribed after a heart attack. It helps prevent blood clots from forming, which is essential for avoiding another heart attack.

Aspirin is a blood thinner (*Antiplatelet*), which means it reduces the ability of *platelets* (tiny cells in the blood) to stick together and form clots which can lead to another heart attack.

Aspirin helps prevent this from happening again. It is often prescribed as a long-term medication, meaning patients may need to take it every day for life unless otherwise advised by their doctor.

While aspirin is generally safe, it can increase the risk of bleeding, especially in the stomach. The most common side effects are indigestion and stomach aches – taking your medicine with food may help reduce this risk. It can produce troublesome heart burns. Aspirin can cause small ulcers to develop in the stomach in some individuals. These ulcers may bleed causing problems for the patient. To lower the risk of stomach ulcers, patients are given "*Enteric-coated Aspirin*" tablets. These tablets are specially designed to dissolve in the intestines rather than the stomach, which helps protect the stomach lining and reduces the chance of ulcers forming. Signs of internal bleeding include blood in stools or unusual bruising of skin. Patients should report any such concerns to their doctor promptly.

Beta-Blockers

Beta-blockers are medications that help reduce the strain on the heart by slowing down the heart rate and lowering blood pressure. This makes it easier for the heart to function and prevents further damage.

Beta-blockers block the effects of *Adrenaline* (the hormone that speeds up the heart), making the heart beat slower and with less force. This lowers blood pressure and reduces the heart's workload. By reducing the workload on the heart, beta-blockers help prevent further damage and reduce the risk of another heart attack. They also help prevent *Arrhythmias* (irregular heartbeats), which are more likely to occur after a heart attack.

Some common beta-blockers include *Metoprolol*, *Atenolol*, and *Carvedilol*. These drugs must be taken daily, with the dosage adjusted based on the patient's response.

Side effects of beta-blockers can include fatigue, dizziness, or cold hands and feet. These often improve as the body adjusts to the medication, but any ongoing concerns should be discussed with a doctor.

ACE Inhibitors and ARBs

ACE inhibitors (*Angiotensin-Converting Enzyme inhibitors*) are prescribed to lower blood pressure and help protect the heart after a heart attack. These medications help relax blood vessels, making it easier for the heart to pump blood throughout the body.

ACE inhibitors block the production of *Angiotensin* II, a chemical that causes blood vessels to constrict. By preventing the blood vessels from narrowing, ACE inhibitors help lower blood pressure and allow blood to flow more easily.

Reducing blood pressure helps lessen the stress on the heart, which is important after a heart attack when the heart may be weakened. ACE inhibitors also help prevent heart failure by protecting the heart muscle from further damage.

Examples of ACE inhibitors include *Lisinopril, Enalapril*, and *Ramipril*. These drugs are usually taken once a day, with dosage adjustments based on blood pressure levels.

The most common side effect of ACE inhibitors is a dry, hacking cough. Other side effects may include dizziness or high potassium levels. If side effects are bothersome, the doctor may switch to a related class of drugs called **ARB**s (*Angiotensin II Receptor Blockers*), which have fewer side effects. For those patients who cannot tolerate ACE inhibitors, the doctors prescribe ARBs which have a similar action but lack the distressing side effect of hacking cough.

Candesartan, Valsartan, Losartan and *Telmisartan* are the commonly prescribed ARBs.

Statins

Statins are a group of drugs used to lower the levels of cholesterol in blood, especially the bad cholesterol (**LDL**). They act on the liver to decrease the production of cholesterol. They are given once daily, usually at night because the body produces more cholesterol at night. The most important side effect of statins is muscle pain, often referred to as *Myalgia*. It is not very common but in some patients, this side effect may be bothersome. The commonly prescribed statins are *Atorvastatin, Simvastatin* and *Rosuvastatin*.

Depending on the presence of other conditions or complications after a heart attack, the patient may be prescribed other drugs like Diuretics or Antiarrhythmic drugs.

Follow-Up

After a heart attack, regular follow-up appointments are essential to ensure that the heart is healing well and to prevent further complications. These visits allow doctors to track progress, adjust medications if necessary, and check for any potential issues.

Follow-up appointments help doctors assess how well the heart is recovering. The doctor will check for any signs of heart failure or *arrhythmias* (abnormal heart rhythms) and make sure that the heart is healing as expected.

As the patient's condition improves or changes, doctors may adjust the doses of medications or add new ones to better control blood pressure, cholesterol, or other risk factors. This is a critical part of ensuring long-term heart health.

These follow-up appointments are an opportunity for patients to discuss any concerns or symptoms, such as chest pain, shortness of breath, or side effects from medications. Open communication with the doctor helps catch any potential problems early.

Common Tests After a Heart Attack

Echocardiogram: This ultrasound test shows how well the heart is pumping and helps assess the damage to the heart muscle. It provides a detailed image of the heart's structure and function. The ejection fraction, which is a measure of the heart's pumping capacity is calculated by the Echo to assess the improvement with medications. This is discussed in detail in in Chapter 12 on *Diagnosis and Investigations*.

Stress test: A stress test evaluates how well the heart handles physical activity. The test checks how well the heart copes with physical activity. During the test, patients may be asked to walk on a treadmill while their heart rate and blood flow are monitored. If the heart responds well, it indicates to the doctor that the patient is likely ready to resume normal activities.

Blood tests: Doctors may perform regular blood tests to monitor cholesterol levels, kidney function, and the effects of medications. These tests help ensure that the treatment plan is working as intended and that the patient's overall health is being maintained.

In the weeks and months immediately following a heart attack, follow-up appointments are typically scheduled every few weeks to closely monitor progress. As the patient's condition stabilizes, these appointments will become less frequent, but regular check-ups every few months remain important to keep the heart healthy.

Long-Term Monitoring Goals

The primary goal of regular check-ups and long-term monitoring is to protect the heart and improve the overall quality of life. By staying on top of heart health and making adjustments as needed, one can reduce the risk of further complications and live a more active, fulfilling life.

Regular monitoring allows doctors to detect potential issues early, such as rising blood pressure, blood sugar or cholesterol levels, before they become major problems. This proactive approach keeps the heart as healthy as possible and prevents further damage.

By keeping risk factors in check and following a comprehensive care plan, patients can maintain a better quality of life. Regular check-ups ensure that any issues are addressed promptly, allowing the patient to focus on living a healthy life without constantly worrying about his heart.

How Patients Can Prepare for Check-Ups

Being prepared for each appointment will help the patient get the most out of the check-ups. By tracking one's symptoms and medications, one can provide the doctor with valuable information that can guide one's care.

It is important to pay attention to how one feels between appointments. Making note of any symptoms like chest pain, shortness of breath, dizziness, or swelling in the legs is important. These symptoms could be signs of heart strain or complications and reporting them to one's doctor helps catch these problems early. Keeping a symptom diary can also help the patient remember the details when talking to the doctor.

One should bring a list of all the medications one is taking to each appointment, including over-the-counter medications and supplements. Any prescriptions from other doctors also should be shown to the cardiologist. It is also helpful to mention any side effects one may have noticed, or difficulties encountered with the treatment plan. For example, if fatigue or dizziness is occurring due to a medication, the doctor may adjust the dose or prescribe an alternative medication. Being open about how one feels helps the doctor make the best decisions for the patient's care.

Post-heart attack care and rehabilitation are essential for recovery and long-term heart health. Cardiac rehabilitation offers a structured program of exercise, nutrition counseling, and emotional support to help patients regain strength, manage risk factors, and build healthy habits. By staying committed to this care plan and making lifestyle changes, patients can significantly improve their chances of living a healthier, more active life after a heart attack.

Key Takeaways

- *Cardiac rehabilitation is a medically supervised program that supports heart health recovery through exercise, nutrition counseling, and emotional support.*
- *It helps patients build healthy habits, manage risk factors, and reduce the likelihood of future heart problems.*
- *Medications like aspirin, beta-blockers, ACE inhibitors, and statins play a critical role in heart recovery and must be taken as prescribed.*

- *Regular follow-up appointments and tests are essential to monitor heart health, adjust treatment, and catch potential issues early.*
- *Psychological support, including counseling and group therapy, is vital for emotional recovery, helping patients cope with anxiety and stress after a heart attack.*
- *Staying engaged in post-heart attack care, following medical advice, and making lifestyle changes can significantly improve long-term heart health and quality of life.*

Chapter 19 LIFESTYLE CHANGES AFTER HEART ATTACK

Surviving a heart attack is a life-changing event that marks the beginning of an ongoing journey toward better heart health. The key to preventing future heart problems lies in adopting essential lifestyle changes. These adjustments—such as embracing a heart-healthy diet, incorporating regular exercise, quitting smoking, and managing stress— play a vital role in your recovery. This chapter provides a comprehensive guide to these changes, offering practical advice on how to improve your heart function and overall well-being. With the right knowledge and support, small, consistent lifestyle changes can lead to a healthier, longer life.

Surviving a heart attack is just the first step in a lifelong journey of managing your heart health. One of the most effective ways to prevent future heart attacks is by making important lifestyle changes. Adopting a heart-healthy diet and incorporating regular exercise into your daily routine are essential in reducing the risk of another heart event. These changes not only help your heart heal but also improve your overall well-being, making you feel stronger and more in control of your health.

A Heart-Healthy Diet

Diet plays a crucial role in heart health, especially after a heart attack. Making smart food choices can help lower cholesterol, control blood pressure, and maintain a healthy weight, all of which significantly reduce the chances of another heart attack. A heart-healthy diet does not just protect your heart but also supports your body's healing and gives you more energy.

A heart-healthy diet focuses on reducing the types of foods that cause clogged arteries, high blood pressure, and excess weight. Instead, it emphasizes eating foods that nourish the heart and help your body function at its best.

Components of a Heart-Healthy Diet

Reducing Unhealthy Fats

Saturated fats and Trans fats are the types of fats that can raise your bad cholesterol (**LDL**) levels. These type of fats are often found in red meat, butter, cheese, and processed foods like cookies and chips. High levels of bad cholesterol can lead to plaque buildup in the arteries, which makes it harder for blood to flow to the heart. Reducing these fats in your diet is important for keeping your arteries clear.

Instead, focus on consuming *Unsaturated Fats*, which are found in foods like olive oil, avocados, nuts, and fatty fish such as salmon. These healthy fats can help improve your cholesterol levels and protect your heart. Unsaturated fats are those that contain one or more double or triple bonds between the molecules. These type of fats are liquid at room temperature in oil form. They also occur in some solid foods. This group can be broken down further into two categories, called *Monounsaturated* fats and *Polyunsaturated* fats.

Nuts like Almonds, Walnuts, Pecans, Hazelnuts, Cashews, Macadamia nuts and Pistachios contain unsaturated fats. Seeds like Chia seeds, Flaxseeds, Sunflower seeds, Pumpkin seeds and Hemp seeds are also rich in unsaturated fats. Soyabeans and Tofu are also rich in unsaturated fats. Including these in a balanced diet can support heart health and offer other essential nutrients for vegetarians.

Limiting Salt (Sodium)

Too much salt in your diet can raise your blood pressure. High blood pressure makes your heart work harder, putting you at greater risk for another heart attack. Salt is often hidden in processed foods like canned soups, fast food, pickles and snacks like salted and fried chips.

To cut back on salt, cook fresh meals at home using herbs and spices to add flavor instead of salt. Reducing your sodium intake can significantly lower your blood pressure and protect your heart. An adult needs only about 1 teaspoon of salt per day (5 grams) to maintain adequate heart health.

Cutting Back on Sugar

Excess sugar, especially from sugary drinks sweets and snacks, can lead to weight gain and increase the amount of unhealthy fats in your blood. Both of these can harm your heart.

Limit sugary foods like cakes, cookies, and soft drinks. Instead, choose natural sweeteners like fruits, which also provide fiber, or use small amounts of honey as an alternative.

Increasing Fiber-Rich Foods

Fiber is a nutrient that helps lower cholesterol by removing it from the body. Foods high in fiber include whole grains like oats, brown rice, and whole wheat bread, as well as fruits, vegetables, and legumes such as beans and lentils. Fiber also helps with weight management by making one feel fuller for longer, preventing overeating and helping to maintain a healthy weight.

Eating More Fruits and Vegetables

Fruits and vegetables are packed with vitamins, minerals, and antioxidants that support heart health and protect against diseases. Aim to include a variety of colorful fruits and vegetables in your meals to get a broad range of nutrients. These foods help reduce inflammation and improve overall heart function, making them key components of a heart-healthy diet. [**Fig 19.1**].

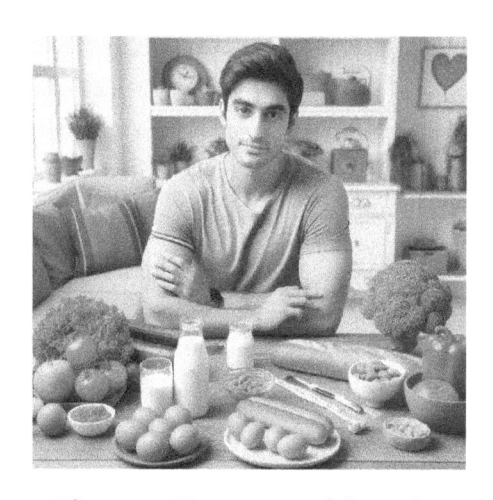

Fig 19.1 Heart Healthy Diet

Figure shows a balance of various foods recommended for prevention of heart disease.

How a Heart-Healthy Diet Helps

By reducing your intake of unhealthy fats, salt, and sugar, you can lower your blood pressure, reduce bad cholesterol, and maintain a healthy weight. These changes are critical in reducing the risk of another heart attack. A balanced, nutritious diet supports your heart's healing process and keeps it strong in the future. Making these dietary changes may seem challenging at first, but small, consistent steps can lead to big improvements in heart health over time.

Regular Exercise And Physical Activity

Along with a healthy diet, regular exercise is one of the most effective ways to strengthen your heart and improve your cardiovascular health after a heart attack.

Physical activity not only helps your heart recover, but it also reduces the risk of future heart problems. By incorporating regular exercise into your routine, you can lower your blood pressure, improve cholesterol levels, and maintain a healthy weight.

After a heart attack, your heart needs to regain its strength. Exercise plays a crucial role in this process by helping the heart pump blood more efficiently and improving overall circulation. In addition, exercise helps manage risk factors such as high blood pressure, high cholesterol, and diabetes. It also has a positive effect on mental health, helping to reduce stress, anxiety, and depression.

Types of Recommended Exercise

Aerobic Exercise

Aerobic exercise is any activity that gets your heart rate up and improves your cardiovascular endurance. This includes activities like walking, swimming, cycling, and light jogging. Playing badminton, tennis or golf are also aerobic exercises. These exercises help your heart use oxygen more efficiently, which lowers blood pressure and reduces strain on the heart.

Experts from the American College of Cardiology recommend aiming for 150 minutes of moderate aerobic exercise each week, which is about 30 minutes per day for five days. If you are just starting out, begin with short, low-impact activities like walking, and gradually increase the intensity and duration of your workouts.

Strength Training

Strength training involves using resistance, like weights or resistance bands, to build muscle. This is important for overall body function and helps with weight management. Stronger muscles can also take some of the workload off your heart during daily activities. Initially, one should start with small weights and slowly build up one's strength. Push-ups, lunges, squats and planks are some of the strength training exercises without the use of weights.

Try to incorporate strength training exercises two to three times per week, but always check with your doctor before starting any strength training routine to ensure it is safe for your heart because strength training increases the heart rate and blood pressure and puts extra burden on your heart.

Flexibility and Balance Exercises

Activities that improve flexibility and balance, such as stretching, Tai-Chi or Yoga, are also beneficial after a heart attack. These exercises help prevent injuries during physical activity and promote relaxation. Flexibility exercises can also ease tension in the body, reducing stress and helping you feel more comfortable and confident as you recover.

How to Start an Exercise Routine

If you are recovering from a heart attack, it is important to start exercising slowly and safely. Begin with light, low-impact activities like walking or gentle cycling. Gradually increase the time and intensity of your workouts as you gain strength and endurance. For many people, cardiac rehabilitation provides a safe, supervised environment to start exercising under medical guidance. Once you are ready to exercise on your own, consult with your doctor to create an exercise plan that is right for you.

Regular exercise helps lower blood pressure, reduce bad cholesterol (**LDL**), raise good cholesterol (**HDL**), and improve blood sugar levels. These benefits reduce the strain on your heart and make it stronger and more efficient. In the long run, staying physically active greatly lowers the risk of another heart attack by keeping your cardiovascular system healthy. It also improves your quality of life, giving you more energy and a better ability to enjoy daily activities.

Lifestyle changes after a heart attack are essential for long-term heart health and preventing future heart problems. By adopting a heart-healthy diet, you can protect your heart and improve overall well-being. Regular exercise, tailored to your individual health needs, strengthens the heart and keeps risk factors like high blood pressure and cholesterol under control. These changes may seem difficult at first, but with persistence and the right support, they can lead to a healthier, longer life.

Quitting Smoking

After a heart attack, making key lifestyle changes is crucial to protect your heart and prevent future heart problems. Two of the most important changes you can make are quitting smoking and reducing alcohol intake. Both smoking and excessive alcohol consumption are major risk factors for heart disease, but by addressing these habits, you can improve your heart health and reduce the strain on your cardiovascular system.

Smoking is one of the most dangerous habits for your heart, and quitting is one of the most effective steps you can take to improve your health. Every cigarette you smoke damages your heart and blood vessels, making it more difficult for your heart to function properly.

How Smoking Affects the Heart

Damage to blood vessels: Smoking damages the delicate lining of your blood vessels (*Endothelium*), making it easier for fat and other substances to stick to the walls of your arteries. This can lead to the buildup of plaque, which can narrow or block arteries, causing a heart attack or stroke.

Increased blood pressure: Smoking raises your blood pressure and heart rate, forcing your heart to work harder than it should. This extra strain weakens the heart over time.

Lower oxygen levels: Smoking reduces the amount of oxygen carried by blood because the carbon monoxide present in cigarette smoke strongly binds to hemoglobin in red blood cells, preventing oxygen from attaching and effectively taking its place, thereby lowering the blood's oxygen-carrying capacity. This compound of hemoglobin with carbon monoxide is referred to as *Carboxyhemoglobin*. This means your heart has to pump harder to deliver enough oxygen to the rest of your body. This increases the workload on your heart, making it more vulnerable to damage.

Benefits of Quitting Smoking

The good news is that the benefits of quitting smoking start almost immediately. Within 20 minutes of quitting, your heart rate and blood pressure start to return to normal levels. After a few days, the oxygen levels in your blood improve, and your heart does not have to work as hard. Over time, the risk of heart disease, stroke, and lung cancer drops significantly. Just one year after quitting, the risk of heart disease is cut in half. After five years, your risk of stroke is similar to that of a non-smoker, and within 15 years, your risk of heart disease is similar to someone who has never smoked.

How to Quit Smoking

Quitting smoking can be challenging for some, but there are many tools and strategies available to help you succeed.

Nicotine replacement therapy: Products like nicotine patches, gum, or lozenges can help reduce cravings and withdrawal symptoms by providing small, controlled doses of nicotine without the harmful chemicals found in cigarettes.

Medications: Prescription medications like *Varenicline* or *Bupropion* can help reduce nicotine cravings and make quitting easier.

Support groups and counseling: Many people find that joining a support group or talking to a counselor gives them the encouragement they need to quit. Cardiac rehabilitation programs often offer these services as part of their comprehensive care.

By quitting smoking, you will reduce the strain on your heart, improve your circulation, and give your body the chance to heal from the damage caused by smoking.

Reducing Alcohol Intake

While moderate alcohol consumption can have some heart benefits, drinking too much alcohol can be harmful, especially for someone recovering from a heart attack. Excessive drinking increases the risk of heart disease, high blood pressure, and other health problems, making it important to limit your intake.

How Alcohol Affects the Heart

Drinking too much alcohol raises the blood pressure, which puts extra stress on the heart and arteries. Over time, this can lead to high blood pressure, a major risk factor for heart attacks.

Excessive alcohol can cause the heart to beat irregularly, a condition known as *arrhythmia*. *Atrial fibrillation* is a common arrhythmia precipitated by binge drinking and it can predispose a person to stroke. This can be dangerous and increase the risk of stroke or heart failure. Alcohol also can depress the contracting function of the heart and hence can prove to be detrimental in patients with a low ejection fraction and heart failure.

Alcohol is high in calories and can lead to weight gain, especially when consumed in large amounts. Carrying extra weight increases the risk of heart disease and places additional strain on the heart.

Often alcohol consumption is accompanied by smoking which aggravates the risk of developing heart disease. Increased alcohol intake is also accompanied by increased food intake which predisposes to obesity.

Guidelines for Safe Alcohol Consumption

If you choose to drink alcohol, it is important to do so in moderation. The general guidelines for alcohol consumption given by the American Heart Association are as follows.

One drink per day for women and two drinks per day for men. One drink is typically defined as 12 ounces of beer, 5 ounces of wine, or 1.5 ounces of spirits. For some people, especially those with certain health conditions, the best choice may be to avoid alcohol altogether. It is always a good idea to discuss alcohol use with your doctor to determine what is safe for you.

Both quitting smoking and reducing alcohol intake offer tremendous benefits for your heart health. These changes help lower blood pressure, improve circulation, and reduce strain on the heart. Over time, making these adjustments can greatly reduce the risk of another heart attack and improve your overall quality of life.

Managing Stress

Stress is a normal part of life and cannot be avoided by anyone, but too much stress, especially after a heart attack, can have serious effects on one's heart. Managing stress and improving one's mental health is essential not only for emotional recovery but also for protecting the heart from future problems.

How Stress Affects the Heart

Stress triggers the release of hormones like *Cortisol* and *Adrenaline*, which can increase the blood pressure and cholesterol levels. Over time, high levels of cortisol contribute to *inflammation* and damage to the arteries. Stress also causes unhealthy behaviors like overeating, smoking, drinking alcohol or avoiding exercise, all of which are bad for the heart.

Stress Management Techniques

Learning how to manage stress effectively is an important part of heart disease prevention. There are several techniques that can help you reduce stress and improve your mental health.

Deep Breathing Exercises

Simple breathing exercises can have a powerful effect on stress levels. Deep, slow breaths help calm the nervous system, lower your heart rate, and reduce blood pressure. These exercises can be done anywhere, at any time, making them a convenient way to relieve stress. This can be repeated 15 – 20 times to feel more de-stressed. The patient is encouraged to concentrate on his breathing while taking in a deep breath and while breathing out.

Meditation and Mindfulness

Practices like *Meditation* and *Mindfulness* help people focus on the present moment and let go of negative thoughts or worries. Regular meditation can reduce anxiety, lower blood pressure, and improve overall emotional well-being. Mindfulness involves paying attention to your thoughts and feelings without judgment, helping you manage stress in a healthier way. These can be practiced regularly, and the habit easily cultivated.

Yoga or Tai Chi

Gentle exercises like *Yoga* or *Tai Chi* combine movement with breathing techniques to reduce stress and improve mental clarity. These activities not only help you stay physically active but also promote relaxation and balance, both mentally and physically. Yoga, in addition offers physical exercises (*Asanas*) which help in improving muscle tone and strength. *Pranayama*, which is a breathing exercise, is also a part of yoga.

The Role of Counseling and Therapy

Emotional recovery is just as important as physical recovery after a heart attack. Many patients experience anxiety, depression, or fear of having another heart attack. Talking to a therapist or counselor can help you work through these emotions and develop strategies for coping with them.

Cognitive-behavioral therapy (**CBT** helps patients reframe negative thoughts and adopt healthier behaviors. CBT is especially helpful for managing stress and anxiety, both of which can affect heart health.

Building a Support Network

Having a strong support system is key to managing stress and staying motivated on the path to recovery. Friends, family, and support groups provide emotional support, encouragement, and accountability. Sharing your experiences with others who understand what you are going through can make a big difference in your recovery. These essential lifestyle changes are needed for improving one's heart health after a heart attack. These changes help to protect your heart, improve your overall well-being, and reduce the risk of future heart problems.

Key Takeaways

- *Making lifestyle changes after a heart attack is essential for long-term heart health and preventing future heart problems.*
- *A heart-healthy diet focuses on reducing unhealthy fats, salt, and sugar while increasing fiber, fruits, and vegetables to support heart recovery and reduce the risk of another heart attack.*
- *Regular physical activity strengthens the heart, improves circulation, and helps manage risk factors such as high blood pressure, cholesterol, and weight.*
- *Quitting smoking and reducing alcohol intake are critical steps in reducing strain on the heart and preventing further heart damage.*
- *Stress management through techniques like deep breathing, mindfulness, and yoga helps reduce the negative impact of stress on heart health.*
- *Building a strong support system, whether through family, friends, or support groups, is key to maintaining motivation and emotional well-being during recovery.*
- *Lifestyle changes may seem challenging at first, but persistence and small, consistent steps lead to long-term improvements in heart health and overall quality of life.*

Chapter 20 PREVENTION HEART ATTACK

Preventing a heart attack is within reach for most people by making heart-healthy choices and managing key risk factors. This chapter highlights simple yet powerful lifestyle changes, such as eating a nutritious diet, staying physically active, and regularly monitoring your health. Understanding the role of cholesterol, blood pressure, and weight management is crucial for lowering the risk of heart disease. Additionally, quitting smoking and limiting alcohol consumption can further protect your heart. Patient education plays a vital role in prevention, as being informed about risk factors and taking proactive steps—such as regular check-ups and managing chronic conditions like diabetes—can significantly reduce the chances of a heart attack. With the right approach, you can take control of your heart health and prevent future complications.

Preventing a heart attack is largely within your control. By adopting healthy habits and managing key risk factors, you can significantly lower your chances of heart disease. Many of the steps for preventing future heart issues are similar to the lifestyle changes already discussed, so we will just revisit these key principles here. It is helpful to review these ideas to reinforce how everyday choices can support heart health and reduce the risk of future problems.

Daily Habits That Lower Your Risk

Making small, consistent changes to your daily routine can have a powerful impact on your heart health. These habits do not require drastic measures, but they do require mindfulness and dedication and a bit of will power.

Healthy Eating

As already discussed, a heart-healthy diet is one of the most effective ways to reduce your risk of heart disease. The food you eat plays a major role in maintaining healthy cholesterol levels, controlling blood pressure, and keeping your heart strong.

Fruits and vegetables are rich in vitamins, minerals, and fiber, all of which are essential for heart health. Fiber helps lower cholesterol, while vitamins and antioxidants protect the heart. Aim to fill at least half your plate with fruits and vegetables, varying the types and colors to get a wide range of nutrients.

Whole grains are present in foods like oats, brown rice, and whole wheat bread and contain high levels of fiber, which helps reduce "bad" cholesterol (**LDL**). Whole grains are also more filling, which can help with weight control—another important factor in heart health.

Not all fats are bad for you. Healthy Fats such as those found in olive oil, avocados, nuts, and fatty fish like salmon, can actually improve cholesterol levels by increasing "good" cholesterol (**HDL**). On the other hand, trans fats and saturated fats, commonly found in processed and fried foods, should be limited, as they can raise LDL and increase the risk of heart disease.

Lean proteins like chicken, fish, legumes, and plant-based alternatives are to be chosen. These are lower in unhealthy fats than red meats, which can contribute to clogged arteries.

Portion control and mindful eating is equally important. It is not just what you eat but also how much you eat that affects your heart health. Overeating can lead to weight gain and obesity, which are major risk factors for heart disease. Eating smaller, balanced meals and paying attention to your hunger and fullness cues can help keep your weight and heart healthy. [See Chapter 19 on *Lifestyle Changes After Heart Attack*].

Exercise and Physical Activity

Staying physically active is another cornerstone of heart disease prevention. Exercise strengthens your heart, improves circulation, and helps manage risk factors such as high blood pressure and high cholesterol.

Moderate exercise like brisk walking, swimming, or cycling for at least 30 minutes a day get your heart pumping and improve your cardiovascular health. Strength training like lifting weights or using resistance bands twice a week can build muscle and improve overall heart function. Strength training also helps maintain a healthy weight, which is critical for heart health.

Incorporating physical activity into daily life is equally important. You do not need to go to the gym to stay active. Small changes, like taking the stairs instead of the elevator, walking instead of driving short distances, or even doing stretches while sitting at your desk, can add up and help keep your heart healthy.

Regular Health Check-ups

Many people may have risk factors for heart disease, such as high blood pressure or high cholesterol, without even knowing it. Regular health check-ups are essential for catching these issues early and taking steps to address them.

Routine check-ups with your doctor is a must to help detect risk factors, such as high blood pressure, high blood cholesterol, diabetes or weight issues, which can contribute to heart disease. Early detection and intervention are key to preventing serious health issues.

Heart disease does not happen overnight—it develops over time due to a combination of risk factors. Controlling these can make a big difference in preventing a heart attack. Let us briefly see how some of the risk factors contribute to the development of heart attack.

> *At 25, Daniel had just married when his father suddenly passed away from a massive heart attack at age 50. His mother, then 60, developed angina and required an angioplasty. With both parents having coronary artery disease, Daniel grew increasingly concerned about his own heart health and consulted a cardiologist.*
>
> *The cardiologist advised him on crucial lifestyle changes to prevent heart disease, emphasizing a heart-healthy diet. A dietitian further tailored his nutritional plan. Daniel was also encouraged to stay physically active, so he joined a tennis club and played five days a week. He limited alcohol to occasional social events, practiced yoga and meditation to manage stress, and prioritized spending time with his family and non-smoking friends. He also made time for hobbies and recreation, leading a balanced and active life.*
>
> *Now, at 65, Daniel reflects on his choices and is grateful to the cardiologist who helped him take proactive steps. Despite a strong family history of heart disease, he has stayed healthy and heart attack-free.*

High Blood Pressure (Hypertension)

Blood pressure indicates the force of blood pushing against the walls of your arteries. When this pressure is too high, your heart has to work harder to pump blood, which can damage your arteries over time.

High blood pressure can often be managed through lifestyle changes, such as eating a low-sodium diet, exercising regularly, and managing stress. In some cases, medication may also be necessary to keep your blood pressure within a healthy range. Uncontrolled high blood pressure can weaken and narrow the arteries, making them more prone to blockages that can cause heart attacks and strokes. Regularly checking your blood pressure and making necessary adjustments to your lifestyle or medications can significantly reduce your risk of heart disease.

High Blood Cholesterol

Cholesterol is a fatty substance in the blood. There are two main types: **LDL** (low-density lipoprotein), often referred to as "bad" cholesterol, and **HDL** (high-density lipoprotein), known as "good" cholesterol. Too much LDL cholesterol can cause plaque to build up in the arteries, leading to blockages that can trigger a heart attack.

You can lower your cholesterol by eating a diet low in saturated fats and high in fiber, exercising regularly, and, if necessary, taking medications like *Statins*. Increasing your intake of foods rich in omega-3 fatty acids (found in fish like salmon and flaxseeds) can help boost your HDL levels, which in turn helps remove excess LDL from your bloodstream.

For people with very high cholesterol or those at high risk of heart disease, medications like statins may be prescribed. These drugs help lower LDL cholesterol levels and reduce the likelihood of plaque buildup in the arteries.

Smoking and Alcohol Consumption

Smoking is one of the most harmful habits for the heart. The chemicals in cigarettes damage the blood vessels, increase blood pressure, and significantly raise the risk of heart disease. Quitting smoking is one of the most important steps a person can take to protect the heart.

While moderate alcohol consumption (one drink per day for women, two drinks per day for men) may have some heart benefits, excessive drinking raises blood pressure and cholesterol levels, increasing the risk of heart disease. Keeping alcohol intake within recommended limits is essential for maintaining heart health.

Chronic conditions, such as diabetes, obesity, and kidney disease, significantly increase the risk of heart disease and heart attacks. By effectively managing these conditions, one can protect the heart and improve overall health.

Diabetes

Diabetes is one of the most critical factors when it comes to heart disease. High blood sugar levels, if not properly controlled, can damage blood vessels and nerves that regulate the heart, increasing the likelihood of heart disease and heart attacks.

Elevated blood sugar causes long-term damage to the lining of the blood vessels (*Endothelium*), making them more prone to plaque buildup (*Atherosclerosis*). This narrows the arteries, restricting blood flow and leading to heart problems, including heart attacks.

How to manage diabetes

Diet: Eating a balanced diet is key. Focus on whole foods, such as vegetables, whole grains, and lean proteins, while reducing your intake of sugary foods and refined carbohydrates, which can spike blood sugar levels.

Exercise: Physical activity plays a crucial role in controlling blood sugar by helping the body use insulin more effectively. Activities like walking, cycling, and swimming are particularly beneficial.

Medications: Many people with diabetes require medications or insulin therapy to manage their blood sugar levels. Following the doctor's guidance on medications is essential for keeping blood sugar within a safe range.

Regular monitoring: Monitoring your blood sugar regularly helps you stay on top of your condition. By keeping blood sugar levels in check, you can reduce the damage to your heart and blood vessels, lowering the risk of heart attacks.

Obesity

Excess body weight strains the heart and contributes to conditions like high blood pressure, high cholesterol, and diabetes, all of which raise the risk of a heart attack. Extra weight, particularly around the abdomen, increases the load on the heart, forcing it to work harder. This can lead to high blood pressure and cholesterol problems, creating the perfect storm for heart disease.

Some weight management tips are given below.

Adopt a balanced diet rich in fruits, vegetables, whole grains, and lean proteins while cutting down on high-calorie, processed foods.

It is not just about what you eat, but also about portion control—eating the right amounts of food can help manage weight effectively. Both the quality and quantity of food matters.

Regular exercise helps burn calories and maintain a healthy weight. Even modest weight loss—just 5-10% of your body weight—can significantly improve heart health.

Other Chronic Conditions

Managing other chronic conditions also plays an essential role in heart attack prevention.

Kidney disease: Kidney problems are often linked with high blood pressure, which can increase the risk of heart disease. Keeping the kidneys healthy through diet, adequate liquid intake, and medications (if needed) can help protect one's heart as well. One should drink at least 2 liters (or quarts) of liquids, per day.

Inflammatory conditions (like arthritis): Chronic inflammation has been linked to heart disease because inflammation can damage blood vessels over time. Properly managing conditions like rheumatoid arthritis through medications, a healthy diet, and exercise can reduce inflammation and, in turn, lower heart disease risks.

Public Health Campaigns & Prevention

Beyond individual lifestyle changes, public health campaigns and initiatives play a significant role in raising awareness and providing resources to prevent heart disease. These efforts have proven successful in reducing heart attack rates and improving public health.

Public Health Campaigns

Public health campaigns aim to educate the public about heart disease, its risk factors, and the steps people can take to prevent it.

Heart disease awareness campaigns: Programs like "*Go Red for Women*" and "*World Heart Day*" work to raise awareness about heart disease. For example, "*Go Red for Women*" specifically targets women, who often experience different symptoms of heart attacks than men, encouraging them to recognize warning signs early and reduce their risk factors.

Educational outreach: Governments and health organizations launch educational initiatives in schools, workplaces, and community centers to promote heart-healthy lifestyles. These efforts encourage better nutrition, more physical activity, and regular health screenings to prevent heart disease.

Healthy Lifestyle Initiatives

Public health initiatives often focus on supporting healthier lifestyle choices that can help prevent heart disease.

Smoking cessation programs: Smoking is one of the most significant risk factors for heart attacks. Many countries have introduced programs that help people quit smoking by providing free counseling, nicotine replacement therapy, and support groups. These programs have been effective in reducing smoking rates and, consequently, heart disease.

Exercise and fitness programs: Community fitness programs, such as park walks, exercise challenges, and free gym access, encourage people to stay active. Regular physical activity reduces the risk of heart disease by improving heart function and helping to manage weight, blood pressure, and cholesterol.

Nutritional guidelines: Programs like the "5 A Day" initiative, which encourages people to eat at least five servings of fruits and vegetables every day, help guide the public towards healthier food choices. Simple and clear guidelines make it easier for people to incorporate heart-healthy habits into their daily lives.

Health Policy and Regulations

Governments also play a crucial role in preventing heart disease through policies that promote healthier environments and reduce risk factors.

Tobacco control laws: Strict regulations on tobacco sales, advertising, and smoking in public spaces have been highly effective in reducing smoking rates and, as a result, decreasing heart disease cases.

Food labeling: Clear nutritional labeling laws that require food companies to display ingredients and calorie counts help consumers make informed decisions and healthy choices. When people are aware of what is in their food, they are more likely to choose heart-healthy options.

<u>Trans-fat bans</u>: Some countries have banned the use of trans fats in food production. Trans fats, which are found in many processed and fried foods, have been linked to heart disease. These bans have led to lower heart attack rates in regions where they have been implemented. Furthermore, the trans-fat content is also included in food labeling which helps people make healthy choices.

Managing chronic conditions and supporting public health initiatives are two powerful strategies in the fight against heart disease. By taking control of health issues like diabetes and obesity, and taking advantage of resources like public health campaigns, a person can greatly reduce the risk of a heart attack. Prevention is always better than cure, and by making small, consistent changes to one's lifestyle and embracing available support, a person can protect the heart for years to come.

Key Takeaways

- *Heart attack prevention is largely achievable through healthy lifestyle choices and managing key risk factors like blood pressure, cholesterol, and weight.*
- *A heart-healthy diet rich in fruits, vegetables, whole grains, and healthy fats helps lower cholesterol, blood pressure, and overall heart disease risk.*

- *Regular physical activity, including moderate exercises like walking and strength training, strengthens the heart and improves circulation.*
- *Regular health check-ups are critical for early detection of risk factors like hypertension and high cholesterol, allowing for timely intervention.*
- *Controlling risk factors such as high blood pressure and cholesterol levels significantly reduces the risk of heart disease and heart attacks.*
- *Quitting smoking and moderating alcohol consumption are key steps in reducing the likelihood of heart disease.*
- *Managing chronic conditions like diabetes and obesity can greatly decrease the risk of heart attacks by improving overall cardiovascular health.*

Chapter 21 MISCELLANEOUS TOPICS

This chapter explores three critical situations where heart attacks can occur or require special precautions: during Pregnancy, during Air or High-altitude travel, and following Non-cardiac surgery. Each

of these scenarios presents unique challenges and understanding them is essential for patient safety and care.

Heart attacks in pregnancy, though rare, are becoming more frequent as more women give birth later in life, making awareness of risk factors and symptoms vital. Air travel and high-altitude activities can stress the heart, especially in individuals recovering from a heart attack, highlighting the need for careful planning and medical consultation. Lastly, heart attacks after non-cardiac surgery often go unnoticed due to the anesthesia or pain medication, stressing the importance of postoperative monitoring. Educating oneself about these risks, can help take proactive steps to safeguard one's health.

Heart Attack and Pregnancy

A heart attack, or *Acute Myocardial Infarction* (**AMI**), happens when blood flow to a part of the heart muscle is blocked, causing damage. While this is rare in women of childbearing age, it can happen, especially as more women over the age of 40 are becoming pregnant. When it does occur during pregnancy, it can pose serious risks for both the mother and baby.

Increasing Incidence of Heart Attacks During Pregnancy

In recent years, heart attacks during pregnancy have become more common, particularly as more women are giving birth later in life. Studies show that heart attacks now happen in about 6 - 10 per 100,000 pregnancies. This is a significant increase compared to earlier studies, which reported 6.2 heart attacks per 100,000 pregnancies (1996).

The timing of heart attacks during pregnancy can vary:

- 20.6% occur during pregnancy itself.
- 23.7% happen during labor and delivery.
- 53.4% take place in the *postpartum* period (after birth).

Risk Factors

Many of the factors that increase the risk of heart attacks in the general population also apply to pregnant women. These include:

- Older age (above 35 years)

- Hypertension (high blood pressure)

- Diabetes

- Obesity

- Smoking

- High cholesterol (*Dyslipidemia*)

- Drug use, particularly cocaine and amphetamines

- Lower socioeconomic status

- Black race, as studies have shown higher incidence rates

- Fertility treatments, which are linked to a higher risk of spontaneous *Coronary Artery Dissection* (a tear in the coronary artery)

Signs and Symptoms

The symptoms of a heart attack in pregnant women are often similar to those seen in the general population. The most common symptom is chest pain or discomfort, which may spread to the shoulders, arms, jaw, or back. Other symptoms include shortness of breath, nausea, palpitations, fainting, and dizziness.

In some cases, women may not experience chest pain, and other atypical symptoms like shortness of breath or nausea may be the only warning signs. Therefore, it is important to monitor these symptoms closely.

Diagnosis

The methods used to diagnose a heart attack in pregnancy are generally the same as those used for anyone else. These include:

- Checking for chest pain as described by the patient.

- Getting an Electrocardiogram (**ECG**) done to note the changes during a heart attack.

- Measuring *Troponin* levels in the blood. A high level indicates that a heart attack has occurred.

Management of Heart Attacks in Pregnancy

Treating a heart attack during pregnancy can be tricky because some treatments may pose risks to the developing baby. Still, managing the mother's health is the top priority, as her well-being directly affects the baby. Here is how heart attacks are usually managed during pregnancy:

Revascularization: This procedure is used to restore blood flow to the heart, often through *Angioplasty*. In some cases, *Coronary Artery Bypass Surgery* may be required.

Medications: Several medications used to treat heart attacks are generally safe during pregnancy, including

Low-dose aspirin (which helps prevent further clots)

Nitrates (used to relax and open blood vessels)

Beta-blockers (which lower blood pressure and reduce the strain on the heart)

Heparin (an *anticoagulant* that does not cross the placenta, making it safer for the fetus)

Fetal Monitoring: The baby's health should be monitored closely, with careful planning for delivery if the mother or baby's condition worsens.

Special Considerations

Radiation: Some diagnostic procedures, like *Angiography* (imaging of the coronary arteries) and *Angioplasty*, require radiation. While this poses a risk to the baby, certain techniques can minimize radiation exposure. If the procedure is needed to save the mother's life, the benefits outweigh the risks.

Delivery: During labor, measures should be taken to reduce stress on the mother's heart. This might include the use of *Epidural Anesthesia* (to reduce pain and stress), oxygen, and close monitoring of blood pressure. The choice between a vaginal delivery and a Caesarian section will depend on the mother's condition.

Medications to Avoid

Certain medications normally used in heart attack are harmful during pregnancy and should be avoided. These are *Statins, ACE inhibitors* and *Fibrinolytic therapy* (clot-busting drugs), which are considered risky during pregnancy. Certain drugs like *Methergine* and *Prostaglandins*, which cause blood vessels to narrow (*constrict*), should also be avoided during labor.

Complications

A heart attack during pregnancy can lead to serious complications. Some of these are:

- Heart failure or Cardiogenic shock which may occur in 38% of cases.
- Ventricular arrhythmias (abnormal heart rhythms) which occur in about 12%.
- Recurrence of angina (chest pain) or heart attack may occur in 20%.
- Decreased heart function, with many women having a *Left Ventricular Ejection Fraction* (a measure of how much blood the heart pumps with each beat) below 40%. In severe cases, it can be below 20%.
- The risk of death from a heart attack during pregnancy is significant, with maternal death rates ranging from 4.5 to 7% in studies. For women who have pre-existing coronary artery disease, it is recommended to undergo stress testing before pregnancy and adjust their medications as needed.

Although heart attacks during pregnancy are rare, they are becoming more common as more women delay childbirth. Managing a heart attack in a pregnant woman requires careful consideration of both maternal and fetal health, with a focus on individualized care. With proper medical attention, many women and their babies can recover well. Still, awareness of the risk factors, symptoms, and complications is crucial for expecting mothers and healthcare providers alike.

High Altitude Travel After a Heart Attack

Recreational activities at high altitudes, such as hiking, skiing, or mountain climbing, pose additional challenges for those with heart disease. The reduced oxygen at higher altitudes makes the heart work harder, and symptoms of heart disease can worsen.

Traveling by air and visiting high-altitude destinations have become common for many people, including those who have experienced a heart attack. However, the body undergoes certain changes at high altitudes, which can be challenging for individuals with heart conditions. After a heart attack, it is essential to be aware of the potential risks associated with air travel and high-altitude activities to ensure a safe trip.

How Altitude Affects the Body

At higher altitudes, the air pressure, oxygen levels, humidity, and temperature decrease. This can lead to *tissue hypoxia* (low oxygen in the tissues), a condition where the body gets less oxygen than it needs. For people with heart disease, this situation can cause:

- Increased heart rate.
- Higher blood pressure.
- More stress on the heart, which has to work harder to pump oxygenated blood to the body.

These changes become significant at altitudes above 2,500 meters (8,200 feet), which is the height at which altitude sickness and other issues can start to develop.

Normal Cardiovascular Response to High Altitude

When a healthy person reaches high altitude, their body makes several adjustments to cope with the lower oxygen levels. The most immediate response is *hyperventilation* (rapid and deep breathing) to try to bring more oxygen into the lungs. The heart also works harder to pump oxygenated blood to the muscles and organs.

For people with a heart condition, this increased workload can sometimes cause problems, especially if they are engaging in physical activities like hiking or skiing at high altitudes.

Special Considerations for Heart Patients

If you have had a heart attack, traveling to high altitudes can increase the risk of complications, such as:

- Angina due to reduced oxygen levels in the atmospheric air.
- *Arrhythmias* (irregular heartbeats), which can be triggered by stress or physical exertion at high altitude.
- Heart failure, especially if the heart is already weakened (low EF) and cannot cope with the increased demands at higher altitudes.

Factors to Consider Before Traveling

Before traveling, particularly to high-altitude areas, individuals with heart conditions should take into account:

- Their baseline health and current heart function.

- The altitude they plan to visit.
- The physical activity they intend to do and the duration of the trip like trekking or skiing.

Managing Altitude Stress

<u>Acclimatization</u>: Take your time to adjust to the altitude. Ascend slowly, and if possible, stay at a lower altitude for a few days before going higher.

<u>Avoid alcohol and heavy meals</u>: Alcohol and large meals can strain your heart more at high altitudes, so it is best to avoid them and eat light before and while in high altitudes.

<u>Watch for symptoms</u>: Be on the lookout for signs of *Altitude Sickness* (such as headaches, nausea, and dizziness), which can mimic or worsen heart symptoms. Carry appropriate medications like *Acetazolamide* (to help acclimate) if advised by your doctor.

High-Risk Groups for High Altitude Travel

Heart failure patients are especially vulnerable. High altitudes can worsen symptoms like shortness of breath and fatigue. Arrhythmias can become more frequent or severe at high altitudes, especially if combined with physical exertion. It is advisable for such patients to avoid high altitude travel as far as possible.

Air Travel After a Heart Attack

Air travel itself is generally safe for most patients after an uncomplicated heart attack, but certain precautions are necessary. The cabin pressure in airplanes is typically maintained at the equivalent of

1,500–2,400 meters (4,900–8,000 feet) above sea level, which can still reduce the amount of oxygen in the air. For people who have had a recent heart attack, this mild drop in oxygen levels might cause discomfort or complications.

When to Fly After a Heart Attack

Let us briefly consider when a person can undertake air travel after a heart attack.

Some patients are classified as *Low-risk patients*. They are those under 65, with a good recovery and no major complications after their heart attack. They can usually fly three days after the event.

Medium-risk patients are those with reduced heart function but no major complications. They should wait for at least 10 days after the onset of heart attack before air travel.

High-risk patients are those with severe damage to the heart or who have major complications. They should wait at least six weeks after a heart attack before flying. They should also confirm with their cardiologist that there is no residual effects of their complications before undertaking air travel.

Safety Tips for Air Travel

- ✓ A Pre-flight assessment is necessary. The patient should talk to their doctor before flying to assess the condition of the heart.
- ✓ They should carry their medications with them in their handbags. They should always carry nitroglycerin or other medications they might need in an emergency. The regular medications

also should be available. A prescription of the doctor should be available with the patient.
- ✓ Supplemental oxygen may be needed by some patients during the flight. If the blood oxygen levels are low, the patient may need to arrange for supplemental oxygen during the flight. This has to be informed to the airlines beforehand.
- ✓ During the flight, the patient should move around and not sit continuously. During long haul flights, the individual should walk or stretch every few hours to prevent blood clots, which can occur during the flights. For this, requesting for an aisle seat is always advisable.

Air Travel and Pacemakers

For people with pacemakers or other implanted heart devices, air travel is generally safe. Airport security scanners may detect pacemakers, but these devices are usually not affected by security equipment. If necessary, patients can request a manual screening.

After a heart attack, air travel and high-altitude trips are not out of the question, but they require careful planning. Always talk to your doctor before making travel plans, especially if you are flying or visiting high-altitude locations. By taking the right precautions, such as waiting for the right time to travel, carrying medications, and knowing your limits, you can enjoy your trip safely.

Heart Attack After Non-Cardiac Surgery

A heart attack can sometimes occur after surgery that is not related to the heart. This happens because the physical and emotional stress of surgery puts extra strain on the body, including the heart. Patients may experience a heart attack due to reduced blood flow to the heart or because of a sudden rupture of plaque in the arteries, leading to blockages.

Interestingly, heart attacks after non-cardiac surgery may not always present the usual symptoms, like chest pain, because patients are often under anesthesia or pain medication. Hence, they may not feel the classical chest pain. Sometimes, the only sign of heart injury is an elevated *Troponin* level in blood (a marker of heart damage) found during routine blood testing after surgery.

How Common is a Heart Attack After Surgery?

Various studies have shown that for adults over 45 who spend at least one day in the hospital for surgery, heart injury after non-cardiac surgery happens in 15 to 20% of cases. This risk increases for older patients and those with existing health conditions.

Risk Factors

Several factors can increase the likelihood of having a heart attack after surgery. Some of these factors are:

Age: Those aged 65 and older are at higher risk.

History of heart disease: If someone has a history of coronary artery disease (narrowing of heart arteries) or peripheral artery disease (poor circulation in the limbs), they are more likely to experience heart problems after surgery.

Diabetes or kidney disease: Both these conditions make it harder for the body to cope with the stress of surgery.

Major blood loss occurring during surgery can reduce the blood flow to the heart and cause a heart attack.

Type of surgery: Emergency surgeries or those involving major organs like liver or kidneys tend to carry a higher risk. Major surgeries in the head and neck, the stomach, intestines and the chest may cause a myocardial infarction during the post operative period.

Signs and Symptoms

Recognizing a heart attack after surgery can be difficult. In many cases, the usual symptoms, such as chest pain, may not be noticeable due to the effects of anesthesia or pain medication. However, some patients may experience symptoms like chest discomfort, shortness of breath, or palpitations due to arrhythmias.

These symptoms can also mimic other complications from surgery, like a *Pulmonary Embolism* (a blood clot in the lungs). Therefore, it is essential to closely monitor patients who are at risk for any evidence of heart attack.

Diagnosis

A heart attack after surgery is usually diagnosed based on two key factors:

1. The patient has had non-cardiac surgery within the past 30 days.

2. There is an elevated troponin level, which indicates damage to the heart muscle.

Other possible causes of increased troponin, such as infections or blood clots have to be ruled out before confirming that the heart is affected. Doctors perform various tests to determine this.

Monitoring After Surgery

Patients with risk factors for a heart attack after surgery, such as older age or a history of heart disease, are often monitored closely in the days following surgery. Doctors may check the Troponin levels at regular intervals—typically 6 to 12 hours after surgery, and then again on the first, second, and third days post-surgery to rule out the possibility of a heart attack.

This careful surveillance helps detect any signs of heart injury early, even if symptoms are not immediately apparent.

Treatment Options

The treatment for a heart attack after surgery depends on the type of heart attack and the patient's overall health.

In a more severe type of heart attack where one of the heart's major coronary arteries is completely blocked, treatment is similar to that of a non-surgical heart attack, including the use of medications to dissolve blood clots and procedures like *angioplasty*. However, if the risk of bleeding is too high after the surgery, doctors may not give medications to dissolve the clots and will alter the treatment accordingly.

When the heart attack is less severe but still dangerous, treatment decisions are often based on the patient's risk of bleeding. If bleeding is not a significant concern, doctors may use medications such as anticoagulants (blood thinners) and beta blockers. They may not plan an immediate angioplasty.

In some cases, doctors may avoid aggressive treatments like angioplasty if the patient is at high risk for bleeding complications and instead continue with conservative treatment giving medications only.

Long-Term Management

For patients who experience heart injury like *ischemia* after surgery but do not have a full-blown heart attack, follow-up care is crucial. These patients should visit their doctor within two weeks after being discharged from the hospital. During this follow-up, the doctor will assess how well the heart is functioning and adjust medications or recommend further tests if necessary.

Heart attacks after non-cardiac surgery are more common than many people realize, especially among older adults or those with pre-existing heart conditions. While the symptoms may not always be obvious due to the effects of surgery, careful monitoring and timely diagnosis are key to ensuring a good outcome.

If you or a loved one is scheduled for surgery and you have any risk factors for heart disease, it is important to talk to the doctor about how to minimize the risk of heart problems. Proper planning and post-surgery monitoring can go a long way in preventing serious complications.

Key Takeaways

- *Heart attacks during pregnancy, while rare, are becoming more common as more women give birth later in life, especially over age 40.*
- *Risk factors for heart attacks in pregnancy include older age, high blood pressure, diabetes, obesity, smoking, and a history of heart disease.*
- *Symptoms of a heart attack in pregnancy can be similar to those in non-pregnant individuals.*
- *Air travel is generally safe after a heart attack for low-risk individuals but should be avoided for unstable high-risk patients.*
- *Physical stress from high-altitude travel can strain the heart, especially in individuals with pre-existing heart disease.*
- *Heart attacks after non-cardiac surgery are more common in older adults or those with existing heart conditions, and symptoms may be masked by anesthesia or pain medication.*
- *Monitoring troponin levels after surgery can help detect heart injury, even if typical symptoms like chest pain are absent.*
- *Treatment, like medicines or Angioplasty, for heart attacks after surgery depends on the severity and the patient's risk of bleeding.*
- *Early follow-up care is crucial for managing heart health after non-cardiac surgery.*

Chapter 22 SUPPORT GROUPS AND RESOURCES

Recovering from a heart attack can be overwhelming, both physically and emotionally, but support groups and resources play a vital role in easing this journey. These groups offer heart attack survivors a safe space to connect with others who share similar experiences, providing emotional support, practical advice, and reassurance. Whether through online communities, local support groups, or professional healthcare teams, the right resources can make a significant difference in your recovery. By accessing these resources, survivors gain a sense of community, valuable insights, and the support needed to navigate life after a heart attack with confidence and hope.

Recovering from a heart attack can be an emotional and physical challenge, but one does not have to go through it alone. There are numerous support groups and resources available to help an individual navigate the recovery journey. These resources not only provide practical advice but also offer emotional support from people who understand what one is going through. Whether through online communities, local support groups, or healthcare providers, finding the right support can make a significant difference in the recovery process.

Where to Find Support After a Heart Attack

Connecting with others who have experienced heart disease, or a heart attack can help you feel less isolated and more confident in your recovery. Support groups, whether online or in person, provide a safe space to share experiences, ask questions, and learn from others who are on a similar journey. Healthcare providers also play an essential role in offering guidance and emotional support.

Online Communities

Online communities offer a convenient way for people recovering from heart attacks to connect with others without leaving home. These virtual spaces allow you to find support whenever you need it and can be particularly useful if you live in a rural area or are unable to attend in-person groups.

Popular Online Platforms

Social Media Groups: Platforms like Facebook host many groups focused on heart attack survivors or those managing heart disease. Members share personal stories, recovery tips, and motivational advice, creating a supportive environment where you can ask questions and share your experiences.

Dedicated Heart Health Websites: Websites such as *Heart.org* (run by the American Heart Association) and *CardiacHealth.org* provide forums where patients can discuss heart health topics and get advice from other survivors or healthcare professionals. Details about heart attack and other heart diseases is also available in these platforms.

Benefits of Online Communities

Convenience and Accessibility: You can access support at any time, from anywhere, without having to travel.

Diverse Perspectives: You will find a broad range of people sharing different experiences, from early recovery to long-term heart health maintenance.

Anonymity: If you prefer privacy, many online platforms allow you to interact anonymously, which can make it easier to share personal concerns.

These online communities can be a valuable source of encouragement and knowledge as you navigate life after a heart attack.

Local Support Groups

For those who prefer face-to-face interactions, local support groups offer the chance to meet others in person, often creating deeper connections and a sense of community. These groups usually meet regularly, providing a reliable source of emotional and practical support during your recovery. Your hospital or your doctor will be able to help you find these groups.

How to Find Local Support Groups

<u>Hospitals and Cardiac Rehabilitation Centers</u>: Many hospitals offer support groups specifically for heart attack survivors. These groups are often led by healthcare professionals, ensuring that discussions are informative and safe.

<u>Community Centers and Non-Profits</u>: Local health organizations or community centers may also host support groups, which often include educational sessions alongside emotional support. These programs are usually free or low-cost, making them accessible to a wide range of people.

Benefits of Local Support Groups

<u>Face-to-Face Interaction</u>: Meeting in person allows for deeper emotional connections and the opportunity to build lasting friendships.

<u>Access to Local Resources</u>: These groups often provide information about local health resources, such as nearby cardiac rehabilitation programs, nutrition workshops, dietitians or exercise classes.

<u>Guidance from Healthcare Professionals</u>: Many local groups involve healthcare professionals who can answer medical questions and provide expert advice on managing your recovery.

Attending a local support group can help you feel more connected to your community and provide a space where you can share both the struggles and successes of your recovery.

Healthcare Providers

Healthcare providers, including cardiologists, nurses, and cardiac rehabilitation specialists, are a cornerstone of your recovery process. Beyond medical care, they offer emotional support and practical advice on lifestyle changes that can improve your heart health.

Types of Healthcare Support

<u>Cardiac Rehabilitation Programs</u>: These structured programs are designed to help you recover physically and emotionally after a heart attack. They often include exercise sessions, nutritional counseling, and mental health support, offering a comprehensive approach to recovery. Patients can find out about these programs from their hospitals or health care providers.

<u>Follow-Up Appointments</u>: Regular check-ups with your cardiologist or primary care provider are essential for monitoring your recovery and adjusting medications or treatment plans. These appointments also offer an opportunity to ask questions about your progress, diet, and emotional well-being.

How Healthcare Providers Support Recovery

<u>Personalized Care</u>: Healthcare providers tailor their advice and treatment plans to your specific condition, ensuring that you get the best possible care.

<u>Referrals to Other Resources</u>: If you need additional support, such as a mental health therapist or a nutritionist, your healthcare provider can refer you to

trusted professionals who specialize in heart disease recovery.

By working closely with your healthcare team, you can ensure that all aspects of your recovery are being addressed, from physical health to emotional well-being.

Family and Friends in the Recovery Process

While professional support is crucial, the role of family and friends in your recovery cannot be understated. Loved ones provide emotional encouragement and practical assistance, which can significantly impact how well you manage your recovery.

Emotional Support

Recovering from a heart attack can be an emotional rollercoaster. You have your ups and downs. Feelings of anxiety, fear, and uncertainty about the future are common, and having a strong support system can make all the difference.

Family and friends can be a source of comfort by simply being there to listen and encourage. Whether you are feeling anxious about your health or celebrating a small recovery milestone, having loved ones who support you emotionally helps lighten the burden.

Encouragement from those close to you can help keep you focused on your recovery goals. Celebrating small victories—like a successful day at cardiac rehabilitation or a change in diet—can make the recovery process feel more manageable. Such encouraging positivity and motivation can be of immense help in recovery and rehabilitation.

Practical Support

In the early stages of recovery, everyday tasks like cooking, cleaning, or managing medications can feel overwhelming. Family and friends can step in to help, ensuring that you have the time and space to focus on healing.

Loved ones can help with shopping, meal preparation, and other daily tasks that may be difficult for you during recovery. Their assistance allows you to rest and concentrate on getting stronger.

In joint families as in India and other Asian countries, often there are close relatives at home who provide support, both physical and emotional for the patients who have had any major illness. The problem arises in nuclear families which is the bane of modernization.

It can be helpful to have someone accompany you to medical appointments. They can take notes, help you remember important instructions, and provide moral support during doctor visits.

Helping with Lifestyle Changes

Making lifestyle changes after a heart attack, such as eating healthier or exercising regularly, is easier when you have the support of those around you.

Family members can join you in adopting heart-healthy habits, such as preparing nutritious meals together or going for walks. Doing these activities as a team can make the changes more enjoyable and sustainable.

Loved ones can also provide gentle reminders to stay on track with your recovery plan, whether that means sticking to your medication schedule or attending cardiac rehabilitation sessions.

It is normal to experience feelings of anxiety or depression after a heart attack, and mental health is a critical part of the recovery process. Family and friends can encourage you to seek professional help if you are struggling emotionally.

If you are feeling overwhelmed, your loved ones can help you find a therapist, counselor, or support group to address your emotional needs. Mental health is just as important as physical recovery, and having someone by your side can help you take that step toward getting help.

Support plays a vital role in the recovery process after a heart attack. Whether through online communities, local support groups, healthcare providers, or the care of family and friends, having people around you who understand your journey can make all the difference. These connections provide emotional comfort, practical help, and the encouragement needed to adopt healthy lifestyle changes. By taking advantage of these resources, you give yourself the best chance for a strong recovery and a healthier future.

Governmental Resources

After a heart attack, navigating the road to recovery can be challenging, both physically and emotionally. Fortunately, there are numerous resources available to heart patients, including programs run by governments and Non-Governmental Organizations (**NGOs**). These resources provide essential support such as financial assistance, educational materials, and community programs to help individuals manage their condition and maintain heart health over the long term.

Governments around the world recognize the importance of supporting heart patients through public health programs. These resources aim to ensure that individuals have access to the necessary treatments and services, regardless of their financial situation.

Medicare/Medicaid

In many countries, heart patients can access health services through government-funded programs like Medicare and Medicaid. In the U.S., for example, these programs provide coverage for various heart-related treatments, including cardiac rehabilitation, prescription medications, and follow-up medical appointments.

Medicare: Primarily for people aged 65 and older, Medicare covers many heart-related services such as hospital stays, cardiac rehabilitation, and doctor visits. Patients recovering from heart attacks can often access rehabilitation programs that help with both physical recovery and lifestyle changes.

Medicaid: Designed to help low-income individuals, Medicaid covers a wide range of healthcare services, including treatment for heart disease. This ensures that those who might struggle to afford care can still receive the medical attention they need.

It is important to check with healthcare providers to understand which services are covered under these programs. Additionally, some countries offer national health programs that provide similar services, ensuring patients can access necessary treatments and follow-up care.

National Health Institutes & Agencies - US

Government agencies such as the *National Heart, Lung, and Blood Institute* (**NHLBI**) in the U.S. provide valuable educational materials and up-to-date research on heart disease. These organizations focus on raising awareness about heart disease, offering prevention strategies, and supporting patients in their recovery.

<u>NHLBI</u>: This institute offers a wide range of educational resources for heart patients, including research updates on the latest heart disease treatments and guidelines for maintaining heart health. Their website provides easy-to-understand information on managing risk factors such as high blood pressure and cholesterol.

<u>International Resources</u>: Many countries have similar government health organizations that offer resources for heart patients. For example, in the UK, the *National Health Service* (**NHS**) provides extensive heart health information, while in Canada, *Health Canada* offers guidelines and support for those recovering from heart conditions.

National Health Institutes & Agencies - India

In India too there are many organizations which provide support to heart attack patients. Some of these are:

Heart Health India Foundation (**HHIF**): In India, the primary Indian organization offering resources and support groups for heart attack patients is the *"Heart Health India Foundation"* (HHIF) - a patient-led organization focused on heart health awareness, support, and advocacy, providing support groups and counseling services for heart patients and their caregivers in India.

Indian Heart Association (**IHA**): This is a prominent organization advocating for cardiovascular health promotion through awareness campaigns and educational initiatives. The *Indian Heart Association* (**IHA**) and Indian Stroke Association (**ISA**) are a cardiovascular health NGO founded by passionate individuals who were personally affected by cardiovascular disease and stroke. The IHA is officially registered in India. The major goal of the organization is to raise awareness about preventative cardiovascular health through a combination of online outreach and grassroots advocacy.

Global Heart Hub: This is an international platform where the *"Heart Health India Foundation"* is listed as an affiliate, providing access to a wider network of heart patient support.

These institutes play a key role in educating the public and heart patients about how to prevent further heart problems and live healthier lives.

Financial Aid Programs

Government programs often include financial assistance to help heart patients cover the costs of treatments, medications, or rehabilitation programs. In the U.S., some patients may qualify for assistance through programs like *Supplemental Security Income* (**SSI**) or *Medicaid*, depending on their income and medical needs.

These financial resources help ensure that cost does not become a barrier to receiving proper care, making it easier for patients to focus on their recovery without added financial stress.

Non-Governmental Resources

In addition to government programs, many non-governmental organizations (**NGOs**) provide crucial support to heart patients. These organizations often offer educational materials, financial aid, and community-based programs to help patients manage their heart health and recover effectively.

American Heart Association (AHA)

The *American Heart Association* (**AHA**) is one of the largest and most respected organizations dedicated to heart health in the United States. It provides a wealth of resources for patients and families, including educational articles, tools for managing heart disease, and patient support networks.

Educational Tools: The AHA offers detailed information on heart disease prevention, treatment options, and lifestyle changes that can improve heart health. Their resources are available online, making it easy for patients to access the latest research and guidelines.

Support Networks: The AHA provides online support groups and local programs where heart attack survivors can connect with others facing similar challenges. These groups offer emotional support and practical advice for managing recovery.

British Heart Foundation (BHF)

For patients in the UK, the *British Heart Foundation* (**BHF**) is a leading resource for heart disease information and support. Similar to the AHA, the BHF focuses on education, patient care, and heart health advocacy.

Research and Campaigns: The BHF supports groundbreaking research into heart disease treatments and runs public campaigns aimed at raising awareness about heart health. They provide clear and accessible information for patients recovering from heart attacks, offering tips on diet, exercise, and medication management.

Patient Support: The BHF also runs support groups and recovery programs that help heart attack survivors connect with others and access the resources they need to recover.

Local Charities and Non-Profits

In many communities, local charities and non-profit organizations offer specialized services for heart patients. These organizations may provide everything from educational workshops to financial assistance for medical expenses.

Community Support: Local organizations often run support groups where heart patients can meet in person to share experiences and recovery tips. These groups create a strong sense of community and can be especially helpful for those who prefer face-to-face interaction over online groups.

<u>Educational Events</u>: Many non-profit organizations also organize health fairs, workshops, or seminars on heart disease prevention, providing valuable information on managing heart health and living a heart-healthy lifestyle.

These non-governmental resources are an important part of the recovery process, offering heart patients a wide range of tools and support options.

Helpful Books, Websites, and Apps

In the digital age, a variety of books, websites, and mobile apps are available to help heart patients manage their condition and stay informed about their health. These resources provide practical advice, health tracking tools, and ongoing education to support long-term recovery.

Books

"Prevent and Reverse Heart Disease" by Dr. Caldwell Esselstyn: This book emphasizes the power of a plant-based diet in improving heart health and reducing the risk of future heart problems. Dr. Esselstyn provides evidence-based recommendations and easy-to-follow tips for adopting a heart-healthy eating plan.

"The Cardiac Recovery Handbook" by Paul Kligfield, MD: This comprehensive guide offers step-by-step instructions for heart attack survivors. It covers everything from physical rehabilitation to emotional recovery, providing practical strategies for regaining strength and preventing future heart attacks.

"Heart: A History" – by Sandeep Jauhar (2018) In this gripping book, best-selling author and cardiologist, Sandeep Jauhar, intersperses his own medical journey with a history of the heart and advances in the field of cardiology.

In addition, books about heart health are also available in the local language in many countries. In India, such books in the regional languages are available in most of the states.

Websites

American Heart Association (www.heart.org): The AHA website is a trusted source for up-to-date information on heart disease. It includes detailed articles on lifestyle changes, treatment options, and tips for maintaining heart health after a heart attack. The site also features tools like heart-healthy recipes and exercise plans.

Mayo Clinic (www.mayoclinic.org): Mayo Clinic's website offers extensive information on heart attacks and heart disease, including patient stories, treatment options, and recovery tips. The site is an excellent resource for those looking to understand their condition and explore the latest research.

Apps

MyFitnessPal: This app helps users track their diet and exercise, making it easier to manage weight, monitor cholesterol, and follow a heart-healthy diet. It's a practical tool for setting and achieving health goals.

Heart Wise Blood Pressure Tracker: For heart patients, keeping track of blood pressure is crucial. This app allows users to record their blood pressure readings and share them with healthcare providers, making it easier to monitor and manage blood pressure regularly.

Support groups and resources are vital in helping heart patients recover after a heart attack. From government programs that provide financial aid and healthcare coverage to NGOs that offer education and community support, there are many ways for heart patients to access the help they need. Books, websites, and apps further assist patients by providing practical tools for managing their condition and adopting healthier lifestyles. By using these resources, heart patients can take control of their recovery and improve their long-term heart health.

Key Takeaways

- *Recovering from a heart attack is both an emotional and physical challenge, but support groups and resources are available to provide crucial help during the process.*
- *Connecting with others through online communities or local support groups can reduce feelings of isolation and provide practical recovery advice.*
- *Online communities offer convenience, diverse perspectives, and the option to participate anonymously, making them accessible to people in various stages of recovery.*
- *Local support groups allow for deeper emotional connections, face-to-face interactions, and access to local healthcare resources.*
- *Healthcare providers, including cardiac rehabilitation programs, play a key role in offering*

personalized care, medical guidance, and referrals to additional support.
- *Family and friends offer essential emotional and practical support, aiding in daily tasks, encouraging healthy lifestyle changes, and providing motivation throughout the recovery journey.*
- *Government and non-governmental organizations offer a range of resources, including financial assistance, educational materials, and access to rehabilitation programs.*
- *Mobile apps, books, and websites provide practical tools for monitoring health, accessing information, and managing lifestyle changes post-recovery.*
- *Emotional and mental health support is as important as physical recovery, and both professional help and community support can help address these needs.*

Chapter 23 THE FUTURE OF HEART ATTACK TREATMENT

Heart attacks have long been a leading cause of death, but exciting advancements in medical research are reshaping how we treat and prevent them. The future of heart attack treatment goes beyond just managing symptoms—it focuses on repairing the heart and preventing future damage. With innovations like stem cell therapy, gene therapy, and advanced medications, we are exploring ways to regenerate heart tissue, reduce scarring, and improve recovery. Additionally, wearable technology and artificial intelligence are enhancing early detection and personalized care. As science progresses, the hope for heart attack patients continues to grow.

Heart attacks have long been a leading cause of death and disability, but advances in science and medicine are providing new hope. Future treatments for heart attacks are not just focused on repairing the damage but also preventing it from happening in the first place. Researchers are exploring ways to harness the body's natural healing powers, develop new drugs, and use cutting-edge technologies to monitor and treat heart conditions more effectively.

Biological Therapies
Using the Body's Own Cells to Repair the Heart

Biological therapies represent one of the most exciting advances in heart attack treatment. These therapies aim to use the body's natural abilities to heal itself, offering new ways to repair heart damage and restore function.

Stem Cell Therapy

Stem cells are special cells that can develop into many different types of cells. In heart attack treatment, they are used to regenerate damaged heart tissue as normally the heart muscle cells cannot regenerate like the liver or skin cells.

After a heart attack, parts of the heart may become damaged or scarred, making it harder for the heart to pump blood. Stem cells are introduced into the heart to help repair or replace this damaged tissue. These cells can transform into healthy heart cells and restore some of the lost function.

The main advantage of stem cell therapy is that it can reduce the amount of scar tissue in the heart and improve its ability to pump blood. This could potentially prevent heart failure, which is a common long-term consequence of heart attacks.

One of the challenges of stem cell therapy is ensuring that the cells reach the damaged area and continue to function as healthy heart cells. Research is still ongoing to improve the effectiveness of this treatment, but early results are promising.

Tissue Engineering

Tissue engineering involves creating new heart tissue in a laboratory setting that can be implanted into a patient's heart to replace damaged sections. Scientists can grow heart cells in the lab, creating small patches of heart tissue. These patches are then grafted onto the damaged areas of the heart, where they integrate with the patient's own tissue and promote healing.

Tissue engineering could help the heart recover more completely after a heart attack by replacing damaged tissue with healthy, functioning cells. In the future, this technology might even lead to the creation of fully functional heart tissue for patients with severe heart damage.

Exosome Therapy

Exosomes are tiny particles released by cells that carry healing molecules. They are tiny sac-like structures that carry proteins, DNA, RNA, and other materials between cell. They can stimulate cells to multiply and differentiate into special cells like heart muscle cells thereby promoting muscle regeneration and repair. They play an important role in reducing inflammation and promoting tissue repair. These particles act as messengers, delivering healing instructions to cells in the heart.

Exosome therapy is a non-invasive treatment with fewer risks compared to traditional surgeries. It holds promise for reducing long-term damage to the heart and helping the heart recover faster after an attack.

Gene Therapy and Its Potential

Gene therapy is another groundbreaking area of heart attack treatment. This innovative approach involves modifying or introducing genes to repair damaged heart tissue or prevent further damage.

Gene therapy involves altering the genetic material (**DNA**) within cells to treat or prevent diseases. Researchers are studying how to deliver healthy genes directly to damaged heart cells. These new genes can help the heart repair itself by boosting the production of proteins that promote cell survival and tissue regeneration.

After a heart attack, many heart cells die, which worsens the damage. Gene therapy can target the genes that control this process, reducing the number of cells that die and keeping the heart functioning better.

Boosting New Blood Vessel Growth

When part of the heart is damaged, the blood supply to that area is often reduced. Gene therapy can stimulate the growth of new blood vessels (a process called *Angiogenesis*) to restore blood flow to the heart. By introducing genes that encourage blood vessel formation, scientists hope to improve circulation in damaged areas of the heart, allowing the tissue to heal more effectively.

One of the main challenges of gene therapy is delivering the genes safely and ensuring they work as intended. There is also the risk of triggering an immune response, where the body attacks the introduced genes or the cells carrying them. As research continues, gene therapy could become a powerful tool for heart attack treatment, helping patients recover more fully by addressing the underlying damage to the heart.

New Drugs to Prevent Heart Damage and Recovery

In addition to biological therapies and gene therapy, new drugs are being developed to prevent heart damage during a heart attack and help patients recover more quickly afterward. Blood clots are the main cause of heart attacks. New drugs are being developed to break up clots faster and more effectively, reducing the amount of damage to the heart.

Inflammation can worsen heart damage after an attack. Researchers are also working on new medications to control inflammation and protect the heart from further injury.

Some new drugs focus on protecting the heart muscle during and after a heart attack. These medications help limit the size of the damaged area and support the heart's ability to pump blood efficiently. Other drugs aim to speed up the body's natural healing process by promoting the growth of new tissue. These medications could be used alongside treatments like stem cells to enhance recovery.

Prevention of Future Heart Attacks

High levels of LDL cholesterol (often referred to as "bad" cholesterol) are a major risk factor for heart attacks. New medications are being tested that can lower LDL levels even further than current treatments, reducing the risk of future heart problems.

Some new drugs focus on stabilizing plaques in the arteries. Plaques that rupture can cause blood clots, leading to heart attacks. By keeping these plaques stable, these drugs prevent rupture of the plaque and lower the risk of another attack.

Latest Advances in Prevention and Management

Prevention and early intervention are key to reducing the risk of heart attacks. Advances in technology and personalized medicine are providing new ways to monitor heart health and prevent heart disease before it leads to an attack.

Wearable Technology

<u>Smart devices</u>: Devices like smartwatches and fitness trackers can monitor your heart rate, detect irregular heartbeats, and even identify early signs of heart problems.

<u>Remote patient monitoring</u>: Doctors can now track patients' heart health remotely using wearable

technology, catching warning signs before a heart attack happens and allowing for earlier intervention.

Personalized Medicine

Personalized medicine tailors treatments to an individual's unique genetic makeup and lifestyle. By understanding a person's genetic risks for heart disease, doctors can create customized prevention and treatment plans. If someone has genetic markers that indicate a higher risk of heart disease, doctors can take preventive steps earlier to lower the risk of a heart attack.

Artificial Intelligence (AI) in Diagnosis and Treatment

Artificial intelligence is being used to analyze medical data more quickly and accurately than humans. This allows doctors to diagnose heart problems earlier and more precisely. AI tools can also help doctors decide on the best treatment options for individual heart attack patients, improving outcomes and reducing complications.

New Guidelines for Lifestyle Changes

Ongoing research is refining what constitutes a heart-healthy diet and exercise plan. New guidelines are helping people lower their risk of heart attacks through improved nutrition and physical activity. Cardiologists are regularly going through various new studies and research to update the guideline for lifestyle changes and treatment of heart attacks.

Quitting smoking is one of the best ways to prevent heart attacks. New tools like nicotine patches, smartphone apps, and medications are making it easier for people to quit and stay smoke-free.

The future of heart attack treatment is full of promise. From biological therapies to cutting-edge technologies like gene therapy and AI, these advancements are transforming how we treat and prevent heart attacks.

Key Takeaways

- *Future heart attack treatments are shifting towards prevention, early intervention, and repairing damage.*
- *Biological therapies, including stem cell and tissue engineering, offer potential to regenerate damaged heart tissue.*
- *Gene therapy holds promise for repairing heart tissue, preventing cell death, and promoting new blood vessel growth.*
- *New drugs focus on clot prevention, controlling inflammation, and improving recovery by limiting heart damage and enhancing tissue repair.*
- *Wearable technology and AI are enhancing early detection, remote monitoring, and personalized treatment.*
- *Personalized medicine tailors treatments based on individual genetic risks, potentially improving prevention and recovery strategies.*

Chapter 24 CARDIAC ARREST AND CARDIOPULMONARY RESUSCITATION

Cardiac arrest is a life-threatening emergency that occurs when the heart suddenly stops beating, cutting off blood flow to the brain and other vital organs. Without immediate intervention, it can lead to death within minutes. Unlike a heart attack, which is caused by blocked blood flow, cardiac arrest is an electrical malfunction of the heart, often occurring without warning. Quick response with cardiopulmonary resuscitation (CPR) is essential to keeping a person alive until professional help arrives.

This chapter educates the public on recognizing the signs of cardiac arrest, such as sudden collapse and absence of a pulse, and explains how to perform CPR—a crucial skill anyone can learn to save lives. By increasing awareness and encouraging CPR and Automated External Defibrillator (AED) training, we can improve survival rates for cardiac arrest and empower more people to take immediate, life-saving action.

Cardiac Arrest

Cardiac Arrest (**CA**) is a life-threatening medical emergency that occurs when the heart suddenly stops beating. The heart's job is to pump oxygen-rich blood to the brain and the rest of the body. When the heart stops, so does the blood flow, leading to a rapid loss of consciousness, and, within minutes, potential brain damage or death.

The distinction between cardiac arrest and heart attack must be understood. Unlike a heart attack—which occurs when a blockage, often due to a blood clot, prevents blood from flowing to parts of the heart—cardiac arrest is an electrical problem in the heart. It happens without warning and can strike anyone, even those without a history of heart disease. Cardiac arrest often leads to death if immediate action is not taken, which is why rapid response with cardiopulmonary resuscitation (**CPR**) is critical.

Sudden CA can occur due to several causes apart from a heart attack. These include *Arrhythmias* (irregular heart rhythms) like *Ventricular Fibrillation*, where the heart's electrical signals become chaotic, and *Ventricular Tachycardia*, where the heart beats too fast. Cardiac arrest can also occur when the heart suddenly stops all electrical activity, causing it to completely halt pumping blood. This is known as "flatlining" (*Asystole*) because, on a heart monitor, it appears as a straight line with no movement. In this state, the heart is unable to send blood and oxygen to the body, making immediate medical help crucial to restore a heartbeat.

Other causes include *Cardiomyopathy* (heart muscle disease), which weakens the heart's ability to pump blood; *Congenital Heart Defects* (present at birth); severe electrolyte imbalances (such as potassium or magnesium), which affect heart function; drug overdose or severe substance abuse; and trauma to the chest, such as from a hard impact or electric shock from appliances or lightning strike.

Cardiopulmonary Resuscitation

Cardiopulmonary Resuscitation, commonly known as **CPR**, is a first-aid technique designed to keep a person alive when their heart stops beating. It involves two main actions:

<u>Chest compressions</u>: Pressing down hard and fast on the chest to manually pump blood to the brain and other vital organs.

<u>Rescue breaths</u>: Breathing into the person's mouth to provide oxygen to the lungs, which helps oxygenate the blood being circulated by chest compressions.

<u>CPR does not restart the heart; its goal is to keep blood flowing until professional medical help arrives.</u> Performing CPR within the first few minutes of cardiac arrest can double or triple a person's chance of survival.

Recognizing Cardiac Arrest: Symptoms and Warning Signs

Recognizing the symptoms of cardiac arrest and acting quickly can mean the difference between life and death. Hence these are elaborated below. The most critical symptoms of cardiac arrest include:

- <u>Sudden collapse</u>: The person may fall to the ground without warning and appear lifeless.

- <u>No pulse</u>: When the heart stops, the pulse disappears. A quick check on the neck or wrist will reveal no pulse beat. Checking the pulse in the side of the neck (*Carotid Artery Pulsation*) is ideal as the wrist pulse may not be readily felt.

- <u>No breathing or abnormal breathing</u>: The person will either stop breathing or have gasping breaths, known as "*Agonal Breathing*." These gasps are not effective breathing and should not be mistaken as normal breaths.

- <u>Loss of consciousness</u>: The person rapidly becomes unresponsive and cannot be awakened by tapping, shouting, or shaking.

If you see someone with these symptoms, it is vital to act immediately. Call emergency services and begin CPR right away. If someone else is nearby, ask them to call emergency services immediately. Every minute without treatment reduces the chances of survival by 7-10%. Time is of the essence.

How to Perform CPR?

Performing CPR is a skill that can save lives, and knowing how to do it correctly is essential. The *American Heart Association* (**AHA**) recommends the following steps for high-quality CPR. You should attend a live demonstration class on CPR or watch videos on how to perform CPR.

Step-by-Step CPR Guide

The following are the steps in performing CPR.

1. Check for Safety

Before starting CPR, ensure that the environment is safe for both you and the victim. Avoid dangerous surroundings, such as heavy traffic or wet areas where electricity may be involved.

2. Check for Responsiveness

Gently tap the person or shake their shoulder and shout -*"Hey, Are you alright?"* to see if they respond. If there is no response, check for breathing and a pulse. If the person is not breathing or only gasping, and you cannot detect a pulse, assume cardiac arrest and proceed with CPR.

3. Call for Help

Dial emergency services immediately or ask someone nearby to call. If you are alone and have a mobile phone, place it on speaker mode and start CPR while you wait for instructions from emergency responders. If an *Automated External Defibrillator* (**AED**) is nearby, have someone bring it to you.

4. Start Chest Compressions

- <u>Positioning:</u> Kneel beside the person (preferably on the right side if you are right-handed), place the heel of one hand in the center of their chest (on the lower half of the breastbone), and place your other hand on top of the first. Interlace your fingers for a firm hold.

- Compressions: Press down hard and fast, at least 2 inches deep, with the goal of compressing the chest about 100-120 times per minute.

- Let the chest rise: After each compression, let the chest fully rise before pushing down again. This helps the heart refill with blood between compressions.

5. Rescue Breaths (if trained)

- If you are trained in CPR, after every 30 compressions, give 2 rescue breaths. Tilt the person's head back slightly to open the airway, pinch their nose closed, and give a full breath into their mouth until you see the chest rise. **[Fig 24.1]**.

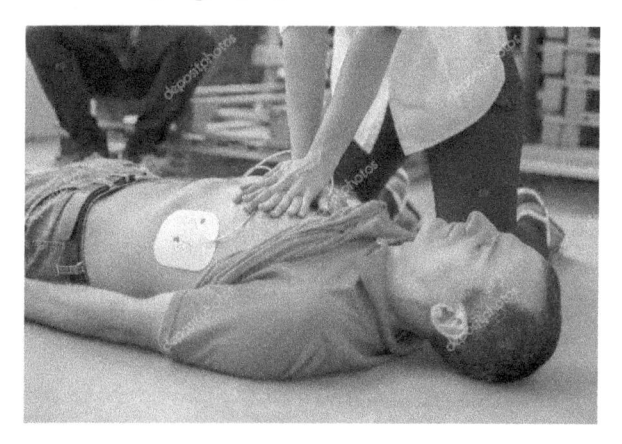

Fig 24.1 CPR in Progress

(Courtesy: Pixelaway / Depositphotos.com)

- If you are not trained, or uncomfortable giving breaths, stick to "hands-only CPR" and focus on chest compressions alone. Hands-only CPR has been shown to be highly effective, especially when administered right away.

6. Continue CPR Until Help Arrives

Do not stop chest compressions unless:

- The person starts moving or breathing.
- Medical professionals arrive and take over.
- An AED arrives and instructs you to pause for a shock.
- You become physically exhausted.

Automated External Defibrillator

An *Automated External Defibrillator* (**AED**) is a portable device that can analyze a person's heart rhythm and, if necessary, deliver an electric shock to help restart the heart. AEDs are designed for public use and can be found in many public places like schools, airports, auditoriums and shopping centers.

Here's how to use an AED:

- <u>Turn on the AED</u>:   Follow the device's audio instructions.

- <u>Attach pads to the chest</u>:   AEDs come with adhesive pads that are placed on the chest according to the diagram on the device.

- <u>Allow the AED to analyze</u>:   The machine will analyze the heart's rhythm and advise whether a shock is needed.

- Deliver a shock: If instructed, press the button to deliver a shock. The shock is meant to *"reset"* the heart's rhythm and allow it to start beating normally again.

- Continue CPR: After the shock, resume chest compressions until help arrives or the person shows signs of recovery.

Using an AED is simple and can significantly increase survival rates when combined with CPR. The American Heart Association estimates that early defibrillation can increase survival rates by 40-60%.

Post-CPR Care
Management After Resuscitation

Once CPR has successfully restarted the heart or after defibrillation with an AED, the person is not out of danger yet. Post-resuscitation care is critical to ensure recovery and prevent further complications. Let us briefly review of what happens after CPR.

Hospital Care

- Stabilization: The first priority is to stabilize the person's heart and breathing. This may include administering medications to control the heart rate and blood pressure.

- Investigating the cause: Medical professionals will perform tests, such as an electrocardiogram (ECG), blood tests, or imaging tests like an echocardiogram (ultrasound of the heart), to determine the cause of the cardiac arrest.

- <u>Preventing further damage</u>: Treatments such as angioplasty or medications to improve heart function may be needed.

- <u>Neurological monitoring</u>: Since the brain is sensitive to a lack of oxygen, doctors will assess brain function to determine if there is any damage. *Therapeutic hypothermia*, where the body is cooled, may be used to reduce brain injury.

- <u>ICU care</u>: Many patients will require time in the Intensive Care Unit (ICU) for close monitoring and support.

Defibrillation
A Key Treatment for Cardiac Arrest

Defibrillation is the process of delivering an electrical shock to the heart to restore a normal rhythm. It is the most effective treatment for certain types of cardiac arrest, such as *Ventricular Fibrillation* (when the heart quivers like jelly instead of pumping blood) or *Ventricular Tachycardia* (an arrhythmia where the heart's ventricles beat too fast).

The AED delivers the shock and can recognize these dangerous rhythms without requiring any input from the user, which makes it a crucial tool in public places. AEDs have been placed in many public places like airports and railway stations. The earlier defibrillation is performed, the greater the chance of survival. For every minute that defibrillation is delayed, the chances of survival decrease by about 10%.

What to Do After Defibrillation?

Even after a shock is delivered, continue performing CPR. The shock from an AED helps reset the heart's rhythm, but it does not always restart the heart immediately. CPR continues to be necessary to support blood flow.

The Importance of CPR and AEDs

Cardiac arrest is a life-threatening event that requires immediate action. CPR, when performed quickly and correctly, can double or even triple the chances of survival. Learning CPR and knowing how to use an AED can make anyone a potential lifesaver.

By spreading awareness about CPR, making AEDs available in more public places, and encouraging more people to take CPR training, we can increase the number of lives saved from cardiac arrest. Quick action and knowledge are key to saving lives in a cardiac emergency. Readers should find out where training in CPR is given in their vicinity and take advantage of these training courses. One never knows when one will need this life-saving procedure.

YouTube Links for CPR

Here are some Links to YouTube videos where you can see CPR being performed. You can watch them and learn the technique of how it is performed. Maybe someday you may save a life!

1. CPR training from the American Heart Association (AHA). Simple demo. Short video.

https://www.youtube.com/watch?v=RNWi4tF9uOA

2. CPR demonstration from the American Red Cross Society.
   https://www.youtube.com/watch?v=VZqG-tcZvfE
3. How to Perform CPR on Adults & Infants in Case of Emergency from the Massachusetts General Hospital by an Emergency Physician. Both Adult and infant CPR are well demonstrated.

https://www.youtube.com/watch?v=BUhUiPeEX-8

4. The British Heart Foundation gives a wonderful training video of CPR in its site.

Bhf.org.uk

Key Takeaways

- *Cardiac arrest is a sudden, life-threatening condition where the heart stops beating, leading to immediate loss of consciousness and potential brain damage or death if not treated promptly.*
- *Cardiac arrest differs from a heart attack, as it is primarily an electrical malfunction in the heart, while heart attacks result from blocked blood flow to the heart muscle.*
- *Immediate action with CPR (cardiopulmonary resuscitation) can significantly increase the chance of survival by maintaining blood flow to vital organs until professional medical help arrives.*
- *Recognizing cardiac arrest is crucial; symptoms include sudden collapse, no pulse, no breathing or gasping breaths, and loss of consciousness.*

- *CPR involves chest compressions and rescue breaths (if trained), with chest compressions alone being an effective method (hands-only CPR) for untrained individuals.*
- *Using an Automated External Defibrillator (AED) in conjunction with CPR can greatly enhance survival rates by delivering an electric shock to restart the heart's rhythm.*
- *AEDs are designed for public use and are found in many places, with simple instructions to guide the user in analyzing heart rhythm and delivering a shock if necessary.*
- *Post-CPR care, including stabilization and neurological monitoring, is essential for the patient's recovery and to prevent further complications.*
- *Defibrillation is the most effective treatment for certain types of cardiac arrest and should be applied as soon as possible for the best outcomes.*
- *Early intervention with CPR and AEDs can double or triple survival chances, emphasizing the importance of public awareness and training in these life-saving techniques.*

Resources & References
Books

1. "***Davidson's Principle and Practice of Medicine***". Ed. Ralston SH et al. 23rd Edition, Elsevier 2018.

2. "***Braunwald's Heart Disease***". Ed. Mann DL et al. 10th Edition. Elsevier Saunders. 2015.

3. "***An Introduction to Electrocardiography***" Leo Schamroth. 8th Edition. 1990. Wiley India Pvt. Ltd. 2013.

4. "***Diabetes Demystified***": Unlock the secrets to Managing Diabetes, Control Blood Sugar, Improve Your Health, and Prevent Complications for a Better Life. (Everyday Health Guide Book 1) Aug. 2024. by Dr. K. V. Sahasranam (Kindle and Paperback) Amazon.com

5. "***High Blood Pressure Demystified***": All-in-One Guide with Practical Advice and Support for Hypertension Patients and Their Families (Everyday Health Guide Book 2) by Dr. K. V. Sahasranam (Kindle and Paperback) Oct. 2024. Amazon.com

6. "***How To Face The Health Challenges While Growing Old***": What Happens to your Heart, Brain, Kidneys, Lungs, Ear, Nose, Throat, Bones & Joints as you age. Get to know Diabetes, Thyroid, Nutritional, and Medical Problems of the Elderly. (Problems Of The Elderly Book 1) by Sahasranam Kalpathy. (Kindle and Paperback) Oct 2022 Amazon.com

7. *"**Old Age Health Challenges and Solutions**":* What happens to your Skin, Gut, Eyes, Teeth, Blood, and Sexuality when you grow old. Know about Psychological, Gynecological, Sleep Disorders, Temperature Regulation, Palliative Care and End-of-Life Care in the Elderly. (Problems of the Elderly Book

2) by Sahasranam Kalpathy. (Kindle and Paperback) Jan. 2023 Amazon.com

References From UpToDate August 2024.

1. **Post-Cardiac Injury Syndromes**: Brian D Hoit, MD Aug 2024.

2. **Left Ventricular Thrombus After Acute Myocardial Infarction**: Gregory Yh Lip.

3. **Suboptimal Reperfusion After Primary Percutaneous Coronary Intervention In Acute St-Elevation Myocardial Infarction**: C Michael Gibson, Ms, Md Joseph P Carrozza, Md Roger J Laham.

4. **Acute Myocardial Infarction: Role Of Beta Blocker Therapy**: Robert S Rosenson, Guy S Reeder, Harold L Kennedy.

5. **Ventricular Arrhythmias During Acute Myocardial Infarction: Prevention And Treatment**: Philip J Podrid.

6. **Perioperative Myocardial Infarction Or Injury After Noncardiac Surgery**: PJ Devereaux.

7. **Treatment And Prognosis Of Cardiogenic Shock Complicating Acute Myocardial Infarction**.   Alex Reyentovich, Holger Thiele.

8. **Acute St-Elevation Myocardial Infarction: Management Of Anticoagulation**.   A Michael Lincoff, Donald Cutlip, Aug 2024.

9. **Left Ventricular Aneurysm And Pseudoaneurysm Following Acute Myocardial Infarction**. James C Fang.

10. **Angiotensin Converting Enzyme Inhibitors And Receptor Blockers In Acute Myocardial Infarction: Clinical Trials**. Guy S Reeder,.

11. **Conduction Abnormalities After Myocardial Infarction.** Peter J Zimetbaum, Joseph E Marine.

12. **Treatment And Prognosis Of Cardiogenic Shock Complicating Acute Myocardial Infarction.** Alex Reyentovich, Holger Thiele.

13. **Clinical Manifestations And Diagnosis Of Cardiogenic Shock In Acute Myocardial Infarction.** Alex Reyentovich, Holger Thiele.

14. **Troponin Testing: Clinical Use** Allan S Jaffe, David A Morrow.

15 **Acute St Elevation Myocardial Infarction: Failed Fibrinolysis.** C Michael Gibson, J Brent Muhlestein,.

16. **Risk Factors For Adverse Outcomes After St-Elevation Myocardial Infarction.** Joseph S Alpert, Peter WF Wilson, Michael Simons, Jeffrey A Breall.

17. **Risk Factors For Adverse Outcomes After St-Elevation Myocardial Infarction.** Joseph S Alpert, Peter WF Wilson, Michael Simons, Jeffrey A Breall.

18. **Acute Myocardial Infarction: Role Of Beta Blocker Therapy.** Robert S Rosenson, Guy S Reeder, Harold L.

19. **Ventricular Arrhythmias During Acute Myocardial Infarction: Prevention And Treatment.** Philip J Podrid.

20 **Left Ventricular Thrombus After Acute Myocardial Infarction.** Gregory YH Lip,

21. **Acute Myocardial Infarction: Mechanical Complications.** Holger Thiele, J Dawn Abbott.

22. **Clinical Features And Diagnosis Of Coronary Heart Disease In Women.** Neha Pagidipati, Pamela S Douglas.

23. **Role Of Echocardiography In Acute Myocardial Infarction.** Neil J Weissman, Bryan Ristow, Nelson B Schiller.

24. **Supraventricular Arrhythmias After Myocardial Infarction.** David Spragg, , FHRS Kapil Kumar.

25. **Electrocardiogram In The Prognosis Of Myocardial Infarction Or Unstable Angina.** Ary L Goldberger.

26. **Clinical Manifestations And Diagnosis Of Cardiogenic Shock In Acute Myocardial Infarction.** Alex Reyentovich, Holger Thiele.

27. **Conduction Abnormalities After Myocardial Infarction.** Peter J Zimetbaum, MD   Joseph E Marine.

28. **Acute Myocardial Infarction And Pregnancy.** Carol A Waksmonski, Anita LaSala.

29. **Silent Myocardial Ischemia: Epidemiology, Diagnosis, Treatment, And Prognosis.** Prakash C Deedwania.

30. **Ventricular Arrhythmias During Acute Myocardial Infarction: Incidence, Mechanisms, And Clinical Features.** Philip J Podrid.

31. **Approach To Patients With Heart Disease Who Wish To Travel By Air Or To High Altitude.** Troy Tuttle, Asif Ali, David Filsoof, John Higgins.

32. **Electrocardiogram In The Diagnosis Of Myocardial Ischemia And Infarction.** Ary L Goldberger, Jordan M Prutkin.

33. **Mechanisms Of Acute Coronary Syndromes Related To Atherosclerosis.** Filippo Crea,   Frank Kolodgie,   Aloke Finn,   Renu Virmani.

34. **Pathophysiology And Etiology Of Sudden Cardiac Arrest.** Philip J Podrid,

35. **Myocardial Infarction Or Ischemia With No Obstructive Coronary Atherosclerosis.** Filippo Crea, Giampaolo Niccoli.

Other References

1. **Acute Myocardial Infarction**: Oren J. Mechanic; Michael Gavin; Shamai A. Grossman.

    https://www.ncbi.nlm.nih.gov/books/NBK459269/

2. **Acute Myocardial Infarction** (MI): ByRanya N. Sweis, MD, MS, Northwestern University Feinberg School of Medicine, Arif Jivan, MD, PhD, Northwestern University Feinberg School of Medicine. Mercke Manual Professional version Feb 2024

    https://www.merckmanuals.com/professional/cardiovascular-disorders/coronary-artery-disease/acute-myocardial-infarction-mi

3. **Myocardial infarction** - Wikipedia:

    https://en.wikipedia.org/wiki/Myocardial_infarction

4. **Atypical Presentations of Myocardial Infarction**: A Systematic Review of Case Reports: Alexander Muacevic and John R Adler. Imran A Khan,1 Habib Md R Karim,corresponding author2 Chinmaya K Panda,2 Ghazal Ahmed,3 and Swatishree Nayak4 . Journal List Cureus v.15(2); 2023 Feb PMC10048062

    https://www.ncbi.nlm.nih.gov/pmc/articles/PMC10048062/#:~:text=Pain%20may%20radiate%20to%20the,common%20atypical%20presentation%2C%20if%20possible.

5. **Heart Attack** - Medically Reviewed by Zilpah Sheikh, MD on September 21, 2023Written by WebMD Editorial Contributors

    https://www.webmd.com/heart-disease/heart-disease-heart-attacks

6. **Heart Attack** - Cleveland Clinic - Heart Attack

    https://my.clevelandclinic.org/health/diseases/16818-heart-attack-myocardial-infarction

7. **Myocardial Infarction in Young Individuals**: A Review Article   Cureus. 2023 Apr; 15(4): e37102   Published online 2023 Apr 4. Alexander Muacevic and John R Adler et al.

https://www.ncbi.nlm.nih.gov/pmc/articles/PMC10166330/

8. **Advancements in Myocardial Infarction Management: Exploring Novel Approaches and Strategies** - Pranav Sachdeva, Kawanpreet Kaur, Saba Fatima, et al. Cureus. 2023 Sep; 15(9): e45578 .

https://www.ncbi.nlm.nih.gov/pmc/articles/PMC10587445/

9. **Heart Attack**   - Medline plus 2017.

https://medlineplus.gov/heartattack.html

10. **Myocardial Infarction.**:   A Maziar Zafari, MD, PhD, FACC, FAHA; Chief Editor: Eric H Yang, MD   et al. May 07, 2019. The heart.org   Medscape

https://emedicine.medscape.com/article/155919-overview

11. **Acute Myocardial Infarction in Young Men Under 50 Years of Age**: Clinical Characteristics, Treatment, and Long-Term Prognosis: International Journal of General Medicine 2021:14 9321–9331 - Authors Gao H, Wang Y, Shen A, Chen H , Li H

Volume 2021:14 Pages 9321—9331 . 4 December 2021

12. **Overview - -Heart attack**: 13 July 2023

https://www.nhs.uk/conditions/heart-attack/

13. **Risk factors for myocardial infarction in women and men**: insights from the INTERHEART study . Sonia S. Anand, Shofiqul Islam, Annika Rosengren, Maria Grazia Franzosi, Krisela Steyn, Afzal Hussein Yusufali, Matyas Keltai, Rafael Diaz, Sumathy Rangarajan, Salim Yusuf on behalf of the INTERHEART Investigators: European Heart Journal, Volume 29, Issue 7, April 2008, Pages 932–940,

https://academic.oup.com/eurheartj/article/29/7/932/482737

14. **Mental Stress–Induced-Myocardial Ischemia in Young Patients With Recent Myocardial Infarction:** Sex Differences and Mechanisms: Viola Vaccarino, MD, PhD, Samaah Sullivan, PhD, Muhammad Hammadah, MD, et al: Circulation - Volume 137, Number 8.

https://www.ahajournals.org/doi/10.1161/circulationaha.117.030849

15. **Health outcomes after myocardial infarction**: A population study of 56 million people in England: Marlous Hall ,Lesley Smith,Jianhua Wu,Chris Hayward,Jonathan A. Batty,Paul C. Lambert,Harry Hemingway,Chris P. Gale. February 15, 2024

https://journals.plos.org/plosmedicine/article?id=10.1371/journal.pmed.1004343

16. **HISTORY - Coronary Heart Disease: From Mummies to 21st Century**: Rachel Hajar, M.D.. Heart Views. 2017 Apr-Jun; 18(2): 68–74.

https://www.ncbi.nlm.nih.gov/pmc/articles/PMC5501035/#:~:text=Coronary%20heart%20disease%20was%20initially,of%20the%20137%20mummies%20studied.

17. **HISTORY - Evolution of Myocardial Infarction and its Biomarkers**: A Historical Perspective: Rachel Hajar, M.D., F.A.C.C. Heart Views. 2016 Oct-Dec; 17(4): 167–172

https://www.ncbi.nlm.nih.gov/pmc/articles/PMC5363097/#:~:text=The%20conventional%20wisdom%20is%20that,is%20caused%20by%20coronary%20thrombosis.

18. **HISTORY - History of Heart Attack: Diagnosis and Understanding** - University of Minnesota.

http://www.epi.umn.edu/cvdepi/essay/history-of-heart-attack-diagnosis-and-understanding/

19. **HISTORY - Acute myocardial infarction — Historical notes**: Rogério Teixeira ,Lino Gonçalves ,Bernard Gersh. International Journal of Cardiology. Volume 167, Issue 5, 1 September 2013, Pages 1825-1834.

https://www.sciencedirect.com/science/article/abs/pii/S0167527312016956

20 **Harold on History | Myocardial Infarction: Evolution in Diagnosis, Care, Prognosis**: John Gordon Harold, American College of Cardiology. Jan 18, 2019.

https://www.acc.org/Latest-in-Cardiology/Articles/2019/01/07/12/42/Harold-on-History-Myocardial-Infarction-Evolution-in-Diagnosis-Care-Prognosis

21. **Historical Perspectives on Management of Acute Myocardial Infarction** - Lee, Z.V., Hanif, B. (2018). Historical Perspectives on Management of Acute Myocardial Infarction. In: Watson, T., Ong, P., Tcheng, J. (eds) Primary Angioplasty. Springer, Singapore. https://doi.org/10.1007/978-981-13-1114-7_1

https://link.springer.com/chapter/10.1007/978-981-13-1114-7_1#citeas

22. **Anatomy, Thorax, Heart:** Ibraheem Rehman; Afzal Rehman. 2023

https://www.ncbi.nlm.nih.gov/books/NBK470256/#:~:text=The%20heart%20is%20a%20muscular,the%20right%20and%20left%20ventricles.

23. **Heart - Overview** Cleveland Clinic:

https://my.clevelandclinic.org/health/body/21704-heart

24. **Heart Anatomy** - Texas Heart Institute:

https://www.texasheart.org/heart-health/heart-information-center/topics/heart-anatomy/

25. **Cardiovascular Disease: A Costly Burden For America Projections Through** 2035 American Heart Association & American Stroke Association (2024).

https://www.heart.org/-/media/Files/About-Us/Policy-Research/Fact-Sheets/Public-Health-Advocacy-and-Research/CVD-A-Costly-Burden-for-America-Projections-Through-2035.pdf

ACKNOWLEDGEMENT

I owe immense gratitude to my family for their unwavering support throughout the process of writing this book. Their encouragement has been invaluable. My daughter, Sandya, has been especially helpful, guiding me through the nuances of computer use and assisting with the text formatting.

My sincere gratitude goes to Prof. R. Krishnan, Senior Physician at Baby Memorial Hospital, Calicut, who generously provided me with invaluable references and resources essential for the creation of this book.

I am also deeply thankful to my colleagues in the author community, who generously assisted me and provided constructive feedback on my previous works. They have been quick to offer advice whenever I faced challenges in my writing.

Special recognition goes to Mr. Som Bathla, my mentor on this journey, and to the members of the Author-Helping-Author (AHA) community, whose guidance has been instrumental in shaping my writing and publishing endeavors.

My teachers in the medical schools where I received my undergraduate and postgraduate training deserve special mention. I have achieved what I have by standing on the shoulders of these stalwarts who taught me the art and science of medicine. My deepest respect and gratitude go to them.

I would like to express my sincere gratitude to depositphotos.com for their outstanding medical illustrations, which have greatly enriched my text.

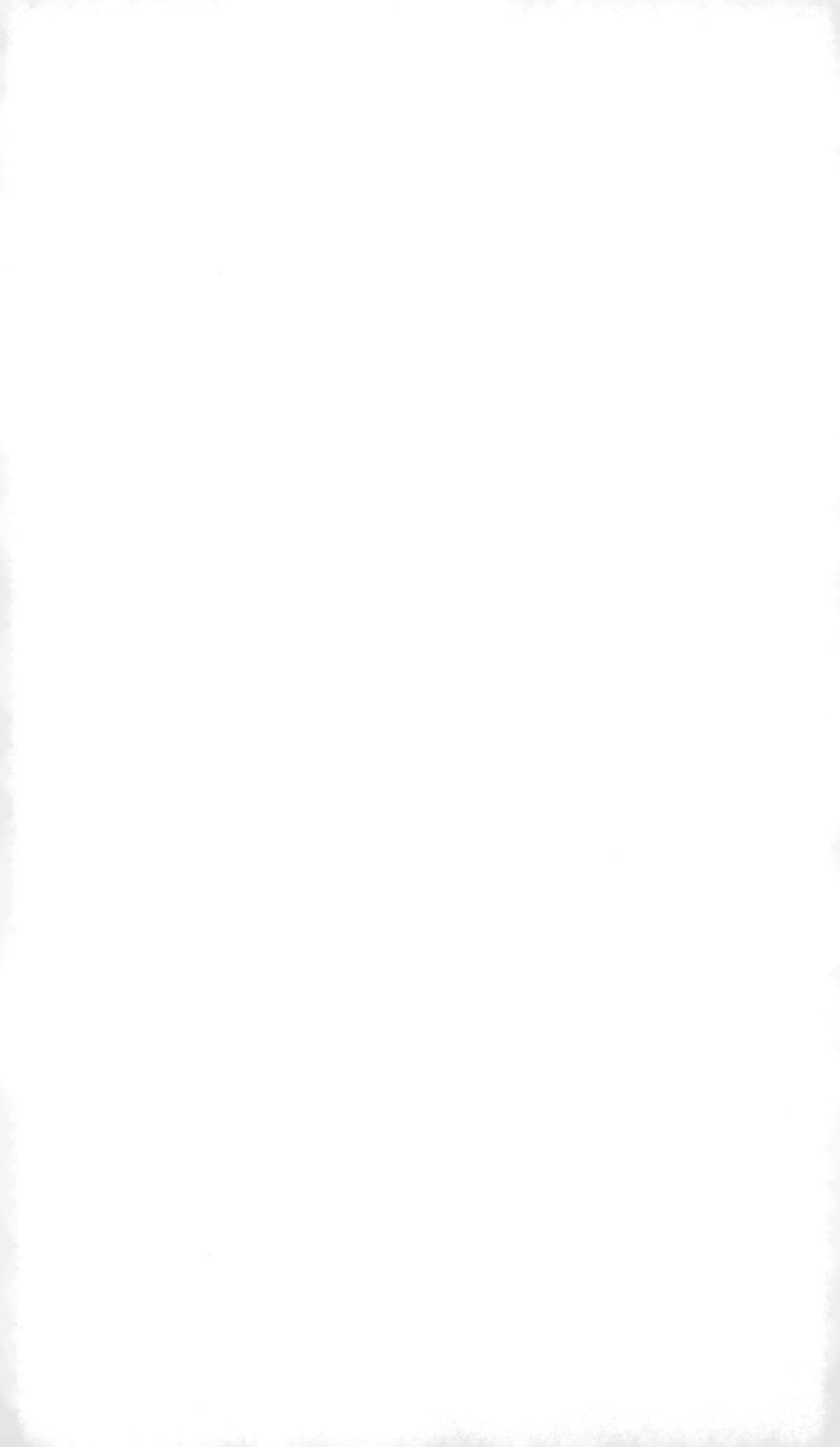

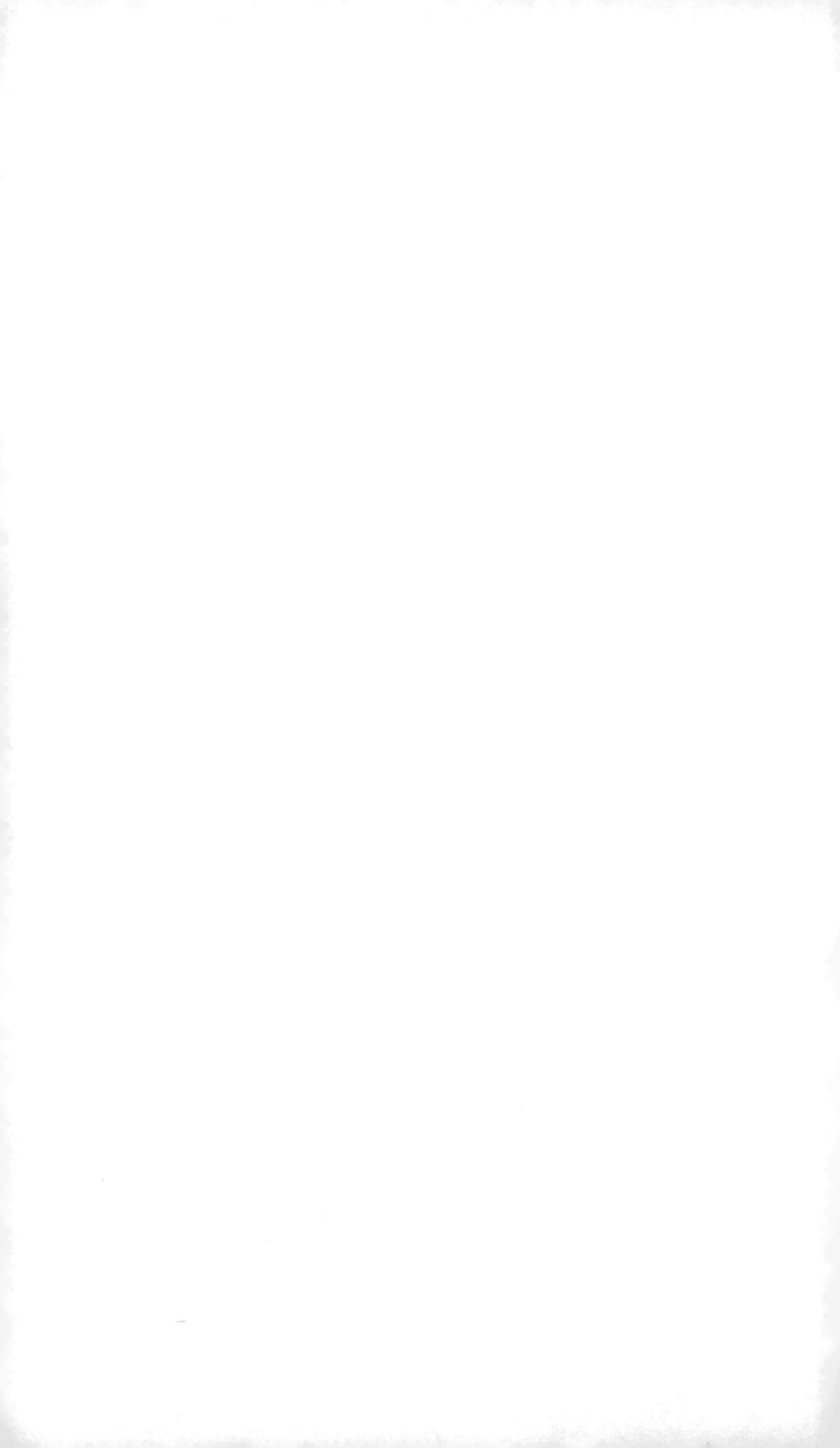